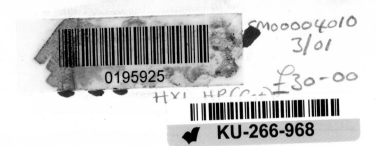
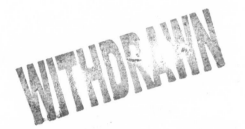

What a Blessing She Had Chloroform

DONALD CATON, M.D.

What a Blessing She Had Chloroform

The Medical and Social Response to the Pain

of Childbirth from 1800 to the Present

Yale University Press   New Haven and London

Published with assistance from the
Mary Cady Tew Memorial Fund.

Designed by Sonia L. Scanlon
Set in Garamond type by Tseng Information Systems, Inc.
Printed in the United States of America

Library of Congress Cataloging-in-Publication Data
Caton, Donald, 1937–
What a blessing she had chloroform : the medical
and social response to the pain of childbirth
from 1800 to the present / Donald Caton.
p. cm.
Includes bibliographical references and index.
ISBN 0-300-07597-9 (alk. paper)
1. Anesthesia in obstetrics—History.
2. Pain—Prevention—History. I. Title.
RG732.C28 1999
617.9'682—dc21 98-36869

A catalogue record for this book is available
from the British Library.

The paper in this book meets the guidelines for permanence
and durability of the Committee on Production Guidelines for
Book Longevity
of the Council on Library Resources.

10 9 8 7 6 5 4 3 2 1

To Cecilia

Sarah, Rachel, Caroline

Audrey, Megan, Emma, Eleanor

and

Margaret Louise

PREFACE

I finished training in 1969, which makes me the product of a system of medical education and practice now almost 150 years old. My career in medicine had begun eleven years earlier, after graduation from college. During the intervening years I had completed medical school, an internship, a residency in anesthesiology, two years of service with the United States Navy, and two years of research training in reproductive physiology. My goal was to teach and practice anesthesia for obstetric patients. At the completion of my training I considered myself as well prepared as any to take on this work.

In 1969 only a handful of anesthesiologists professed having a special interest in obstetrics. Traditionally, obstetricians had managed the pain of labor themselves. With the advent of new drugs and techniques, more patients with medical problems, and the increasing risk of malpractice suits, obstetricians preferred turning the task of anesthesia over to specialists. Obstetrics fascinated me, and I enjoyed the various branches of science on which it draws: physiology, embryology, anatomy, and endocrinology. Working in a university hospital allowed me to pursue these interests in conjunction with practice and teaching.

To my surprise, many women did not want my help. Some were afraid of anesthesia and preferred to accept the pain of childbirth. A larger and more vocal group thought anesthesia was an unnecessary, even dangerous intrusion into childbirth. Many of the nurses working in the labor and delivery unit agreed with them, and no arguments, lectures, clinical studies, or experimental data could change their minds. For them, obstetric anesthesia was not a medical matter but a personal and social issue.

I soon learned that the social issue was surprisingly complex. Ostensibly, it sprang from protest movements of the 1960s, which continued through the 1980s. Large segments of the population demonstrated for civil rights and the environment and against the government and the Vietnam War. People distrusted chemicals, drugs, the government, and virtually anyone in a position of authority, including physicians. These were only part of the problem, however. Many of the women were dealing with another, even larger issue, one with a much longer history. Childbirth, it seemed, had forced them to confront the "problem of pain," as C. S. Lewis called it—its meaning, its role in the life of the individual, and its significance for society. Listening to my patients, I realized that their reactions to childbirth encompassed an extraordinarily wide range of historical and contemporary values.

This book is the result of my attempt to understand and explain the reactions of women to the pain of childbirth. It has three parts. The first part (Chapters 1–5) describes the history of the medical management of the pain of childbirth, a history that begins in 1847 with the first use of a modern anesthetic for labor. This event occurred in the midst of a period of tremendous change in medical theory and practice. Within one generation, physicians threw out a system of practice that had been in effect for almost two millennia, replacing it with the system we use today. The early history of obstetric anesthesia must be viewed, therefore, in the context of the development of modern medicine. Physicians had to learn to use anesthesia, but they also had to learn to think and act like scientists. Readers without a scientific bent may take heart. These early times were filled with colorful people. Insofar as their quirks and personalities influenced medical practice, I have included them in this narrative.

The second part of the book (Chapters 6–10) deals with social reactions to childbirth. Coincident with the revolution in medical practice was a major change in social thought. During this period many people discarded ideas they had once thought essential to the functioning of society, among them the belief that pain and suffering are inevitable components of life. This change in thought was the beginning of an important humanitarian movement in which society created new institutions to deal with poverty, torture, mental illness, imprisonment, and slavery. At the same time, women began to react differently toward childbirth pain, a trend that accelerated during the feminist and suffrage movements of the late nineteenth and early twentieth centuries.

The third part of the book (Chapters 11–12) deals with the interaction between medical practice and social values. I have tried to show the adjustments that have occurred between physicians, who tend to deal with the pain of childbirth as a scientific problem, and patients, who tend to view childbirth as a social, economic, political, or personal problem. Although patients have often felt thwarted by physicians, in truth they have had far more influence on practice than they have realized, and this, I believe is an important lesson for both physicians and patients. Although historically physicians discovered what *could* be done, it was ultimately the patients who decided what *would* be done. Two physicians who had the greatest impact on obstetric anesthesia, James Young Simpson and Grantly Dick Read, were the least scientific but had an extraordinary grasp of the mood of their patients. Each defied the medical establishment and in the process became a folk hero. Most of this material appears in Chapters 11 and 12, but it is insinuated throughout the book. The interplay between "scientific truth" and "social values" occurs throughout medical history. This interplay may be so apparent in obstetrics because of the highly charged connotations of childbirth for the woman, her family, and the community.

I want to define some words that you will find in this book and that you may have encountered elsewhere. *Anesthesia* describes absence of sensation. *General anesthesia* describes the same state accompanied by a loss of consciousness, as normally occurs with exposure to ether, chloroform, and nitrous oxide—the first anesthetics. In talking about anesthesia, the words *nerve block, local, regional, spinal,* and *epidural* refer to loss of sensation without loss of consciousness. Cocaine was the first drug used to achieve "local anesthesia."

The word *analgesia* describes an absence of pain, a state usually obtained with general or local anesthesia. Physicians may use other drugs to diminish pain—aspirin, for example, or opioids, a large group of drugs that includes codeine, morphine, Demerol, and heroin. There are several differences between *anesthetics* and *analgesics.* Most significant is the amount of pain relief that they provide. Anesthetics are capable of abolishing all of the body's normal response to pain. In contrast, analgesics only diminish this response. Thus, codeine will alleviate but not eliminate the pain of a toothache. In normal doses, analgesics may sedate, but rarely do they cause a patient to become unconscious.

Other words often associated with the relief of pain are *narcotics, anodynes, sedatives, tranquilizers,* and *sopo-*

rifics. All refer to applications that may alter a patient's state of consciousness. Only narcotics and anodynes are analgesic. Sedatives, tranquilizers, and soporifics do not relieve pain. Though stuporous, patients treated with these types of drugs still respond to painful stimuli with an increased heart rate, altered respiration, or withdrawal of a limb.

The complex nature of pain tends to confuse technical differences among different groups of drugs. For example, although tranquilizers do not alleviate pain, they may be helpful in its treatment because fear and anxiety often accompany pain. Similarly, although narcotics are not sedatives, patients do sleep better once their pain has been relieved. The historical connotations of many of these words lend further complications. To physicians accustomed to their use, however, each word has a special meaning.

A note about sources. Documenting the medical issues was easy. The scientific and medical literature pertinent to these problems has been part of my professional life for more than thirty years. Documenting social history was more difficult. Fortunately I had considerable help from books and articles. The social implications of clinical practice have been a popular subject for medical historians for several years— almost to the point that many have ignored scientific and medical ideas that shaped practice. To supplement these historical sources, I drew heavily from literature—not medical literature but real literature. Poets, playwrights, and novelists, a group unusually sensitive to the mood of the public, have often dramatized the social and medical issues, particularly when they were in conflict. Many of their works were a rich source of commentary. I assume that a book or essay became popular and lasted only if it reflected the values of its readers.

In the last chapter, I review the historical trends and

describe manifestations of historical values and conflicts in today's patients. In addition, I offer some observations about the nature of pain and suffering and the reactions of people to them. I hope this material will appeal to women who are facing childbirth and to the physicians, nurses, and others who care for them. Finally, I hope that readers will have as much fun reading this book as I had preparing it.

ACKNOWLEDGMENTS

I am deeply indebted to many people. John Sommerville and Frederick Gregory had many important suggestions about the presentation of historical material. Mary A. Thomas shared many ideas and insights about Grantly Dick Read and made useful suggestions about the organization of the material. Lynn Dirk and Pauline Snider gave invaluable editorial assistance. Patrick Sim and Sally Graham of the Wood Library-Museum of Anesthesiology in Chicago suggested many new references and then helped me to find them. Sally Bragg and Christopher Lawrence made my two visits to the Wellcome Institute of Medicine both pleasant and productive. I am grateful to innumerable staff members of the Institut für die Geschichte der Medizine in Vienna, the Wellcome Institute for the History of Medicine in London, the Library of Yale University, and the Medical Library of the University of Florida. Dr. Nicholas M. Greene gave invaluable help by providing my first opportunity to explore medical history and by offering encouragement and critical comments at all stages of my work. I am also grateful to Jean Thomson Black and Mary Pasti of Yale University Press for their encouragement and their generous help in the preparation of this manuscript.

Several organizations gave partial support for the project: the Josiah Macy Foundation, the Wellcome Trust, and the National Institutes of Health. Lippincott publishers and the editors of *Anesthesiology* graciously gave their approval to use portions of five of my papers originally published in that journal:

> Obstetric anesthesia: the first ten years (33:102-109, 1970)
>
> Obstetric anesthesia and concepts of placental transport: a review of the nineteenth century (46:132-137, 1977)
>
> The secularization of pain (62:493-501, 1985)
>
> The poem in the pain (81:1044-1052, 1994)
>
> "In the present state of our knowledge": early use of opioids in obstetrics (82:779-784, 1995)
>
> Who said childbirth is natural? The medical mission of Grantly Dick Read (84:955-964, 1996)

I am especially grateful to Margaret Masters Good, my secretary, who provided invaluable help in so many ways, from obtaining references to preparing "just one more final draft." My greatest debt, however, is to my wife, Cecilia, who has suffered with and by me through the whole project— listening, editing, encouraging, consoling, and criticizing as needed.

Thanks, too, to Queen Victoria—her response to the news that her oldest daughter, Vickey, had been anesthetized for childbirth gave me the title for this book.

PART I

Physicians and the Pain of Childbirth

"The Head of Jove and the Body of Bacchus"

James Young Simpson and the Beginning of

Obstetric Anesthesia

James Young Simpson, who will ever be remembered as the

discoverer of the pain annulling power of chloroform, was

born in the year 1811, at a period when there was room for a

hero in the practice of the healing art in the British Islands.

—H. Laing Gordon, *Sir James Young Simpson,* 1897

"The position of woman in any civilization is an index of the advancement of that civilization; the position of woman is gauged best by the care given her at the birth of her child." So wrote H. W. Haggard in 1929. If so, western European society made a significant advance on January 19, 1847, when James Young Simpson, a Scottish obstetrician, administered diethyl ether to facilitate delivery of a child to a woman with a deformed pelvis. This is the first known administration of anesthesia for childbirth. On the same day, Simpson received notice of his appointment as Queen Victoria's "Physician in Scotland." A comment to his brother shows the relative value that Simpson placed on the two events: "Flattery from the Queen is perhaps not common flattery, but I am far less interested in it than in having delivered a woman this week without any pain while inhaling sulphuric ether. I can think of naught else." Considering everything that had happened to Simpson that day, his lapse in syntax is understandable.[1]

Simpson recognized the medical and the social implications of his achievement and what it offered women. Descriptions of labor pain have always been heartrending. The author of the Book of Jeremiah, for example, notes the "cry of a woman in travail, the anguish of one bringing forth her first child, gasping for breath, stretching out her hands crying 'Woe is me!'" Homer in *The Iliad* refers to "the sharp sorrow of pain [that] descends on a woman in labour, the bitterness that the hard spirits of childbirth bring on." Comments from modern authors are no less moving. The novelist Doris Lessing describes how "the warning hot wave of pain swept up her back [and] she entered a place where there was no time at all. An agony so unbelievable gripped her that her astounded and protesting mind cried out it was impossible such pain should be. It was a pain so violent that it was no longer pain, but a condition of being." The poet Sylvia Plath described labor as a "long, blind, doorless and windowless corridor of pain waiting to open up and shut her in again," and the poet Judith Hemschemeyer calls the delivery "that moment when I knew if I pushed I would die and if I didn't push I would die but it would still be inside me." Simpson's innovation offered women an opportunity to avoid an extremely painful experience.[2]

Ether: A Tale of Three Cities

The sequence of events that prompted Simpson to administer ether had started just a few weeks earlier. On October 16, 1846, William Thomas Green Morton, a dentist in Boston, gave the first successful public demonstration of a modern anesthetic for surgery in a room at the Massachusetts General Hospital, now preserved as the "ether dome." News of Morton's success traveled quickly. Within two weeks a description appeared in the *Boston Medical and Surgical Journal.* One man who had witnessed the event, Dr. Jacob Bigelow, wrote to Francis Boott, an expatriate American physician practicing in London. By December 19 Boott and James Robinson, a dentist, had designed an apparatus to administer ether and had used it for a tooth extraction. Two days later in London the surgeon Robert Liston used ether to anesthetize a man for amputation of an infected leg. Simpson knew Liston, having worked for him as a wound dresser when Simpson was in medical school. On December 26 Simpson traveled to London to speak with Liston about ether. Presumably Simpson used this information three weeks later when he anesthetized his obstetric patient in Edinburgh. Not a person to hide his accomplishments, Simpson promptly described the delivery in an article that appeared in March 1847.[3]

The interval between Morton's demonstration of ether for surgery and Simpson's application of it for obstetrics barely exceeded three months. Given the ship-borne communications of the day, physicians disseminated the news and acted on it with extraordinary speed. Simpson, too, responded quickly. He and the others hardly had time to assimilate the information, much less test it, before they began to use ether in their practices.

The incorporation of anesthesia into medical practice appears especially rapid when compared with the slow and methodical testing procedures of today. The difference reflects changes in medicine over the past century and a half. Contemporary medicine is a highly technical multidisciplinary field. Physicians undergo extensive training in science, mathematics, statistics, and the critique of scientific papers. Not only do private and government organizations oversee and regulate all aspects of medical care, but the public also questions drugs and testing procedures.

In 1847, however, training in science and in critical analysis was not part of medicine. Medicine as we now know it had hardly taken shape. Physicians were only a few decades from medical theories inherited from the ancient Greeks. Physiology, pharmacology, and pathology were in their infancy, and the bacterial origin of disease was unknown. Except for a handful of progressive schools, medical education consisted of an unstructured apprenticeship or a stint reading medical textbooks. No rules or conventions governed the testing of drugs. Anyone could tout the miracles of a new therapy to a public that had little experience evaluating such

claims. Anesthetics were among the first potent drugs that
physicians or the public had to evaluate.

Events in Boston, London, and Edinburgh presented a
formidable challenge. For the first time physicians had an
effective way of obliterating pain, something everyone had
ostensibly wanted for centuries. But physicians suddenly felt
compelled to ask whether it was wise to use that power.
As they soon would learn, various answers had social and
religious implications. The use of anesthesia for obstetric
pain proved to be especially vexatious, and physicians and
patients responded in every way possible. Some called anesthesia "God's gift." Others considered it a needless danger
and even an abomination. These differences were eventually
reconciled, but not without rancor and debate.

Simpson was an active participant in the debate. He not
only introduced anesthesia to obstetrics but almost single-
handedly effected its use, and for this he deserves great
credit. Medical historians who assert that no other physician
could have done this as quickly or as well cite his professional stature and extraordinary personality as factors critical in his success. No less important was the character of the
times. In 1847 all elements of society, including the medical
profession, were in the midst of tremendous change. The
prevailing mood was buoyant and optimistic, and there was
an eagerness to implement new ideas. The incorporation
of anesthesia into obstetric practice represents a fortuitous
confluence of the right person, the right place, and the right
social climate.

Simpson's Life

Many events in Simpson's early life prepared him for the role
of medical innovator. Born on June 7, 1811, in Bathgate, a

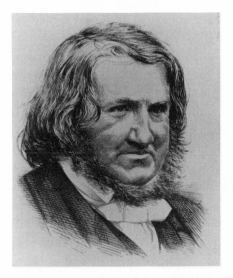

James Young Simpson (1811–1870).
Courtesy of the Wood Library-Museum
of Anesthesiology, Chicago.

small town on the coach route between Edinburgh and Glasgow, Simpson was the eighth and last child of David and Mary Jarvis Simpson. His father was a baker whose business never quite achieved success. His mother died when James was nine years old, so his care devolved on the eldest sibling, a sister.[4]

James studied in a village school directed by a man named Taylor, a teacher of some talent who prepared several of his students to become university professors. On the strength of Simpson's early performance and his aptitude for study, his family pooled their resources so that James might obtain more education—a common practice among poor Scottish families. At age fourteen he began studies at the University of Edinburgh, eighteen miles from home.

Simpson undertook the arts curriculum at the university,

a standard course of study that included rhetoric, mathematics, literature, Greek, and Latin. He enjoyed this work and later put it to good use, but he did not excel. During his first year of study, a friend and fellow student from Bathgate, John Reid, took Simpson to anatomy lectures by Robert Knox, curator of the museum of the College of Surgeons. Knox, a gifted speaker and popular teacher, was an "extra academic" lecturer. Students could satisfy degree requirements by attending courses given by either university faculty or by such extra academics—teachers who taught privately. Stimulated by Knox's lectures, Simpson started formal medical studies in 1828. His professors included the obstetrician James Hamilton, the pathologist John Thomson, and Robert Liston, an extra-academic surgeon from whom Simpson later learned about ether anesthesia.

After finishing his medical coursework in 1830, Simpson assisted at a local dispensary while preparing his doctoral thesis. The thesis, "Death from Inflammation," attracted the attention of his former pathology professor, John Thomson, who offered Simpson work as an assistant. When Thomson later suggested that he consider a career in obstetrics, Simpson studied seriously in that field. Having slept through most of Hamilton's lectures as a student, Simpson sat through them again, this time more motivated to listen than to sleep. On completion of his formal coursework, he visited medical centers in Paris, Liège, Brussels, Ghent, London, and Oxford, a common pattern of postgraduate study. After the tour, he returned to Edinburgh to begin obstetric practice and to lecture as an extra-academic teacher.

Simpson's reputation as an exceptional physician and teacher grew quickly. When he was elected president of the Royal Medical Society in 1835, his inaugural address drew favorable comments, was printed in the *Edinburgh Medical and Surgical Journal,* and was subsequently translated into French, Italian, and German. But in spite of a heavy clinical load, Simpson's income remained limited, and he felt professionally unsatisfied.

In 1839 James Hamilton resigned from the university chair of midwifery. Even though Simpson's youth, limited professional experience, lack of reputation, unmarried status, and modest social origins all militated against success, the twenty-eight-year-old Simpson applied for the post. Professional obscurity may have been the most significant impediment. Local success notwithstanding, Simpson was unknown outside the city. Edinburgh merchants depended on the "medical trade" for income. The economy of the city depended in part on the reputation of the medical school and its professors to attract students and wealthy patients from other cities and countries. Responsibility for selection of Hamilton's replacement lay with the lord provost, the city magistrates, and the thirty-three members of the town council, not with a university committee. Involvement of the town council probably worked in Simpson's favor, for most members of the medical faculty supported his opponent, Philip Syme. In fact, Syme campaigned against Simpson in support of another candidate.

Simpson worked aggressively for selection. He solicited more than seventy testimonials from physicians who knew him, aided no doubt by the contacts made during his study tour of European clinics—Simpson was not easily overlooked or forgotten. Simpson quieted criticism of his bachelorhood by proposing marriage to Jessie Grindlay, whom he had known for several years. Jessie was a distant relative and the daughter of a Liverpool merchant who had helped Simpson during his training. To demonstrate his preparedness for the university post, Simpson collected books, anatomic casts, illustrations, medical equipment, and other paraphernalia that he would need to teach midwifery—more than seven hundred items in all—and set his new wife to the task of cataloging the material for presentation to the town council. Simpson told the council that his lack of reputation did not matter, because, once appointed, he would quickly rise to the top of his profession. Faced with such bravado, the council apparently chose to overlook Simpson's youth, inexperience, and lower-class origins. On February 14, 1840, the council elected him "Professor of Medicine and Midwifery and of the Diseases of Women and Children" by a margin of one vote. He was twenty-nine years old and in serious debt from costs accrued in competing for the post. But the status of a university appointment virtually ensured professional success and financial solvency. It also gave Simpson a platform from which he might be heard and seen.

Simpson used the opportunity that came with his appointment to advantage. An indefatigable worker and an excellent publicist, he quickly became one of the best-known physicians in western Europe. He wrote many professional papers, devised new surgical procedures, and developed a set of obstetric forceps that is still used frequently today. In addition, he became a prominent spokesman for improvements in medical practice, medical education, hospital design, and new methods of care for patients with tuberculosis and leprosy. He also discovered the anesthetic properties of chloroform. Because this very potent, rapidly acting agent was much easier to administer than ether and less irritating to the lungs and throat, it gained in favor. Its popularity lasted for more than half a century before physicians recognized its potential to destroy the liver. Besides pursuing his career in medicine, Simpson developed an interest in archaeology, lecturing and writing on a variety of topics. Most important, Simpson's clinical reputation attracted patients from England and the continent and helped to keep Edinburgh hotel rooms filled with patients and the city solvent. At the time that Simpson administered the first obstetric anesthetic, he was near the crest of his career.

Simpson the Man

Simpson had a memorable appearance. A contemporary wrote:

> The chair was occupied by a young man whose appearance was striking and peculiar. As he entered the room his head was bent down and little was seen but a mass of long tangled hair, partially concealing what appeared to be a head of very large size. He raised his head and his countenance impressed one as that of a pale face, massive bent brows from under which stone eyes now piercing as it were to your innermost soul, now melting into almost feminine tenderness. And finally, now his mouth would seem the most expressive feature of the face. Then his peculiar rounded soft body and limbs, as if he had retained the infantile form in adolescence. All this presented an ensemble which even if we had never seen it again, would have remained indelibly impressed on our memory.

Similarly impressed but less respectful, another acquaintance quipped that "Simpson had the head of Jove and the body of Bacchus." Even as a child, Simpson's head size had attracted attention. The fascination continued after death. Reflecting a Victorian preoccupation with phrenology, Simpson's obituary included detailed measurements of his brain, which weighed fifty-four ounces.[5]

Simpson's personality also impressed observers. Contemporaries described him as a man of immense physical energy, enthusiasm, and charm, mighty passions and strong beliefs. Some said that in conversation he had an almost hypnotic effect on both men and women. Simpson inspired great loyalty and affection but also great enmity. One lifelong adversary was Philip Syme, the famous surgeon who had opposed Simpson's appointment to the medical faculty. The feud continued unabated to their deaths.[6]

Simpson's home in Edinburgh was a center of excitement and activity. No one, including the family and staff, ever knew how many he would bring home as last-minute dinner guests. He enmeshed friends and acquaintances in his projects. When searching for an anesthetic to replace ether, he invited friends for dinner and then asked them to test compounds, which he would pass around the table. According to one story, he recognized the anesthetic potential of chloroform, a very strong agent, when he awoke after one such incident and found himself on the floor flanked by guests who were as unconscious as he had been.[7]

When Simpson died in 1870, many considered him to be among the most famous and influential physicians of the century. More than thirty thousand people filled the streets of Edinburgh for his funeral, according to newspaper reports. The two thousand people who followed the hearse included representatives from the university, from the Colleges of Physicians and of Surgeons, and from other professional societies. An announcement in the *Medical Times Gazette* read, "One of our greatest men has passed from amongst us; Simpson is dead!" The *Lancet* published "Prometheus," a poem dedicated to Simpson.[8] Friends placed a memorial in Westminster Abbey, commissioned a larger-than-life statue to be erected on Princess Street, and attached a brass plaque to the door of his house at 52 Queen Street. The memorial, statue, house, and plaque remain.

Medical Education in the Early Nineteenth Century

Simpson rose to prominence at a time when medicine had little basis in science. Professional advancement depended on rhetoric, political alignments, and the ability to repel the verbal and even physical attacks of rivals. A contemporary described Simpson's Edinburgh as "a city where controversy and partisanship attended portentous developments, where elections [were] fierce battles, and their intervals, times not so much of peace as of preparation."[9] In this atmosphere, Simpson competed and thrived.

Chief among Simpson's advantages was his education. In 1825, when Simpson began his university studies, education in Scotland had a long tradition of excellence. Social historians attribute this excellence to the Reformed religious tradition, which made each person responsible for his or her own soul. Clerics believed that personal knowledge of the Scriptures enabled people to recognize the importance of God's word and to act accordingly. The church, therefore, placed high value on original and independent thought and encouraged development of state support of education. Village schools offered excellent training, as did the universities, which cost the student relatively little to attend. Higher education was accessible to even students with little money, like Simpson. As a result, the people of Scotland were among the best educated in western Europe.[10]

Medical education in Scotland also excelled. By 1800 four of its cities boasted schools: Glasgow, Saint Andrews, Aberdeen, and Edinburgh. What distinguished these medical schools from their English counterparts was their association with a university, medical curricula that emphasized scholarship, the low cost to the student, and freedom from a religious test for matriculation. Most medical schools in England were associated with a hospital or clinic. Their teaching was utilitarian but not inspired. Oxford and Cambridge did have medical programs, but they were small and weak, for these universities gave more emphasis to preparing students for church or government service than for a medical profession. Nor were scholarship and investigation part of the tradition in English medical schools. Original work was most likely to be done by practicing physicians, such as Richard Bright and Thomas Sydenham; or by curious pastors, such as Stephen Hales and Joseph Priestley.[11]

The high quality of medical education in Scotland attracted many students from outside the country. At a time when Edinburgh awarded almost two hundred doctor of medicine degrees each year, Cambridge awarded fewer than four, and Oxford's medical school was virtually defunct. The year that Simpson administered the first obstetric anesthetic, 1847, more physicians practicing in England had a degree from a medical school in either Scotland or the continent than from one in England.[12]

Of the four medical schools in Scotland, most people thought Edinburgh to be preeminent in instruction. It had been founded in 1726 by five former students of the Leiden physician Hermann Boerhaave, one of the most influential medical educators in Europe. The reputation and influence of the Edinburgh Medical School reached its zenith in the last decades of the eighteenth century. Graduates staffed a disproportionate number of teaching posts in medical schools and biology departments in England, Ireland, and Scotland. Edinburgh graduates also had an enormous influence on medical education in America. William Shippen (1736–1808) and John Morgan (1735–1789) founded the first medical school in America, at the University of Pennsylvania. Benjamin Rush (1745–1813), also an original member of the faculty at the University of Pennsylvania, signed the Declaration of Independence and wrote America's first textbook on mental illness. Samuel Bard, a New York physician, founded King's College Medical School, the second medical school in the colonies; and David Hosack started the College of Physicians and Surgeons, the medical school of Columbia University.[13]

Appointment to the Edinburgh faculty gave Simpson one more important advantage, tenure in the oldest and possibly the most prestigious chair of midwifery in the world. Founded in 1726, the chair grew in reputation with each of its incumbents. This growth in status was important, for obstetrics was not a highly regarded specialty in 1847. That honor went to medicine, although surgery was fast closing the gap. Even though family practitioners delivered a high proportion of babies, particularly in cities, medical schools in England did not require a course in obstetrics for graduation. Scottish medical schools did, however, and their graduates influenced the development of the specialty in other countries. Shippen, for example, made a course in obstetrics part of the original medical curriculum at the University of Pennsylvania and taught it himself. Appointment to the chair of midwifery at Edinburgh, therefore, gave Simpson a bully pulpit, which he used to establish obstetric anesthesia.

Simpson's Contribution to the Acceptance of Anesthesia

In 1847 anesthesia needed strong advocates. Although some physicians recognized its potential immediately, many harbored doubts. Criticism fell into two categories. The first concern involved the medical significance of pain—whether pain was a deleterious and unnecessary part of disease or whether it was a necessary component of healing. The second concern was the safety of anesthesia, the nature and magnitude of the risks associated with its use, and the worth of taking those risks. In light of the information available at the time, both concerns were reasonable. Physicians had little information to guide them.[14]

Simpson, unlike many others, had no doubts. To him pain was unnecessary and destructive. In an early paper he quoted the second-century Greek physician Galen: "Pain is useless to the pained." Simpson also pointed out the inconsistency of those who argued that the relief of pain with ether might be detrimental. He reminded his colleagues that physicians had used opium for centuries to relieve pain and suggested that no reasonable distinction could be drawn between the effects of a remedy that was swallowed and the effects of one that was inhaled.[15]

Simpson even claimed that anesthesia itself could be beneficial, suggesting that surgical patients recovered faster if they had been anesthetized. To support this contention, he published statistics showing that the mortality rate associated with amputation of the thigh decreased from 50 to 25 percent when patients were anesthetized. He attributed this difference to the ability of anesthesia to protect the patient from the nervous shock that often occurred during surgery without anesthesia:

> I have already shown, from evidence of statistical returns, that some of the graver operations of surgery are so much less fatal in their results when patients are operated on under anaesthesia, and consequently without any pain, than the same operations were formerly,

when patients were submitted to all the agonies of the surgeon's knife in their usual waking state. The prevention of pain in surgical operations is, in other words, one means of preventing danger and death to those operated on: the saving of human suffering implies the saving of human life. And what holds good in relation to pain in surgery holds good in relation to midwifery.[16]

Simpson made a great leap when he equated the pain of childbirth with the pain of surgery. Unfortunately his claim that anesthesia had a beneficial effect was far less well substantiated for obstetrics than for surgery. He said that "the mortality accompanying labor is regulated principally by the previous length and degree of the patients' sufferings and struggles," but he gave no supporting arguments or evidence. Similarly, it was pure supposition for him to write "as in surgery, [ether's] utility is certainly not confined to the mere suspension and abrogation of conscious pain, great as by itself such a boon would doubtless be, but in modifying and obliterating the state of conscious pain, the nervous shock, otherwise liable to be produced by such pain . . . is saved to the constitution, and thus an escape gained from many evil consequences that are too apt to follow in its train."[17] Inasmuch as Simpson had anesthetized only six women when he wrote this, it is difficult to imagine what experience warranted this conclusion. Closer examination of the data from his own institution might have given him cause for thought. Even though maternal mortality was high by today's standards—one death for every 134 deliveries in Simpson's own unit—it was nowhere near the 50 percent mortality that he had reported for leg amputations without anesthesia. Statistics would have been more convincing than rhetoric.

Simpson acknowledged the need to evaluate the safety and side effects of anesthesia. In an early paper he had written: "A careful collection of cautious and accurate observations will no doubt be required before inhalations of sulfuric ether is adopted to any great extent in the practice of midwifery. It will be necessary to ascertain its precise effects both upon the action of the uterus, and on the assistant abdominal muscles; its influence, if any, upon the child: whether it gives a tendency to hemorrhage or other complications; the contraindications peculiar to its use; the most certain modes of exhibiting it; the length of time it may be employed, etc." In this one passage, Simpson astutely predicted the problems with anesthesia that would occupy obstetricians for the next century and a half. Simpson, however, did not act upon his own advice. He continued to extol the benefits of anesthesia without offering further proof. He said that he never had "observed any harm whatever, to either mother or infant" but that he had seen "no small amount of maternal suffering and agony saved by its application."[18]

It is hard to say how much longer women would have had to wait for anesthesia had it not been for Simpson's advocacy. He had the wit to recognize the potential of anesthesia, the courage to apply it to an old medical problem, a reputation that made others listen, and the persistence to see that his innovation took hold. He was aided by his charisma, a keen eye for publicity, and a talent for sensing the mood of patients and winning them to his cause.

In 1847 success seemed close at hand. Writing about ether to a fellow obstetrician, Charles D. Meigs of Philadelphia, almost a year after his first use of the gas, Simpson said, "In midwifery most or all of my brethren in Edinburgh employ it constantly. . . . In London, Dublin and elsewhere it every day gains converts to its obstetric employment; and I have no doubt that those who most bitterly oppose it now will be yet, in ten or twenty years hence, amazed at their own professional cruelty. They allow their medical prejudices to smother and overrule the common dictates of their profession and of humanity." [19] Ironically, Meigs became one of the loudest and most effective opponents of obstetric anesthesia. No doubt Simpson would have been more amazed if he could have foreseen the hostility of some women to obstetric anesthesia one hundred years later.

CHAPTER TWO

"A Cup of Circe"

The Opposition to Obstetric Anesthesia

The favorable results in surgery have been appealed to,

as triumphant proofs of the success and safety of this drug,

and as a cogent reason why it should be equally used in

midwifery. But the circumstances attending administration

of chloroform for the performance of a surgical operation,

and for the prevention of labor-pain are widely different.

—William Featherston Hough Montgomery,

Objections to the Indiscriminate Administration

of Anaesthetic Agents in Midwifery, 1849

Very different from Simpson in both background and appearance was Charles Delucina Meigs, a major opponent of obstetric anesthesia. Simpson came from a poor Scots family; Meigs, an American, came from a socially prominent, financially secure, and well-educated family. Simpson was corpulent, his head unusually large, and his hair flowing; Meigs had a spare frame, sallow complexion, thin lips, and short, straight hair. Simpson had a mellifluous, almost hypnotic voice, Meigs a squeaky monotone. Simpson has been revered in history; Meigs, often reviled. Yet Meigs, no less than Simpson, was well known, articulate, tenacious, and passionate in the defense of his ideas. Like Simpson, Meigs was a prolific writer and a teacher of great power and influence.

Charles D. Meigs typified the prevailing attitude of nineteenth-century obstetricians toward childbirth. He believed that childbirth was a natural process and should proceed at its own pace with the least possible intervention by midwives or physicians. To him, anesthesia was a dangerous and unnecessary medical intrusion.

Popular support for Meigs's attitude was waning, however. Even as Meigs and Simpson argued the merits of anesthesia for obstetrics, physicians were exploring the use of new methods to manage labor, ergots (the alkaloidal stem parts of certain funguses) to induce or intensify contractions, and forceps to facilitate delivery. The controversy surrounding anesthesia was only an aspect of a larger movement within the specialty of obstetrics. Meigs was a strong spokesman for conservative practices and, for a time, was an effective foil to Simpson.

Charles D. Meigs, Opposition Leader

The Meigs family, originally English, had lived in Connecticut since 1647. Charles's grandfather, "Return" Jonathan Meigs, was a minor Revolutionary War hero who earned his nickname by sailing from Connecticut to Long Island to raid the British and then returning safely. An uncle was the first governor of Ohio. Charles's father, Josiah, a Yale graduate and lawyer, had been a clerk for the city of New Haven and a co-founder of the *New Haven Gazette.*[1]

The year that Charles was born, 1792, the Josiah Meigs family was living on the island of Saint George, Bermuda, where Josiah was working as a proctor in the Courts of the Admiralty. Unfortunately, two years later Josiah's attempt to defend an American seaman who had been taken illegally by the British precipitated an unpleasant incident, which caused the family to leave. They returned to New Haven, where Josiah was appointed professor of mathematics and philosophy at Yale by Ezra Stiles, president of the university and a family friend. Seven years later Josiah left Yale because of political differences with Timothy Dwight, Stiles's successor. The family moved to Athens, Georgia, where Josiah became the first president of that state's newly founded college.

Charles Meigs attended the University of Georgia, graduating in 1809.[2] For several years he served as an apothecary and leecher in a town near Augusta under the preceptorship of Dr. Thomas Kendall. Meigs then moved to Philadelphia, where, in 1817, he earned a degree in medicine from the University of Pennsylvania. The next year he received an honorary medical degree from Princeton. Meigs and his wife, the daughter of a Philadelphia merchant, moved to Atlanta, then a small town, where he began practice. Because Meigs's wife abhorred slavery, they returned to Philadelphia

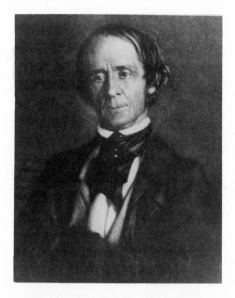

Charles D. Meigs (1792–1869). Courtesy
of the Harvey Cushing/John Hay
Whitney Medical Library, Yale University.

after just two years. One son, Montgomery, graduated from
West Point, became an Army engineer, and later served in
the Union Army as quartermaster general during the Civil
War. Montgomery Meigs also designed several buildings in
Washington, D.C., supervised one of the early renovations
of the Capitol, and chose the site for the Arlington National
Cemetery. Another son, John Forsyth Meigs, and a grandson,
Arthur Vincent Meigs, were physicians known for their con-
tributions to pediatrics.[3]

While in practice, Charles lectured on midwifery in the
Philadelphia Association for Medical Instruction, a private
school. He was also a founding editor of the *North Ameri-*

can Medical and Surgical Journal and translated two French textbooks into English, Velpeau's *Elementary Treatise on Midwifery* and de l'Isere's *Treatise on the Diseases and Special Hygiene of Females.* In 1835 Meigs applied for appointment to the chair of midwifery at the University of Pennsylvania but, after a hotly contested campaign, lost to Hugh L. Hodge. He published his first textbook, *The Philadelphia Practice of Midwifery,* in 1838. In 1841 he was appointed to the chair of midwifery of Jefferson Medical College in Philadelphia. Publications continued: *Woman, Her Diseases and Remedies* appeared in 1847, and *The Science and Art of Obstetrics* in 1849 — its fifth edition was released in 1867, two years before Meigs's death.

In spite of his austere appearance and unimposing voice, Meigs was highly regarded by his patients, students, and colleagues. Many considered him one of the most influential American physicians of the nineteenth century. Like Simpson, however, he had the capacity to arouse great enmity. In Meigs's case, the hostility continued long after his death — and not without reason, for he had an extraordinary talent for making highly inflammatory statements. Feminists today, for example, criticize the condescending tone of his textbooks. Among other things, he said that a woman "has a head almost too small for intellect and just big enough for love" and that the pain of labor had never been great enough to prevent women from having more children. His comments relating intelligence to head size illustrate the intense interest in phrenology prevalent at that time.[4]

Meigs aroused even more lasting enmity when he placed himself on the wrong side of a major nineteenth-century medical issue. Specifically, he doubted the contagious nature of "childbed fever," a lethal infection of the uterus that occurs during childbirth. Even before the discovery of bacteria, physicians suspected that they themselves might be responsible for transmitting some "poison" from one pregnant woman to another. Oliver Wendell Holmes, anatomist and the father of the chief justice, suggested this possibility in 1843. His paper, based on a few observations and many assumptions, had relatively little impact until Meigs criticized it. The publicity created by Meigs's comments gave Holmes the opportunity to write an impassioned rebuttal, which did attract attention. History proved Holmes right—eventually Louis Pasteur isolated and identified the bacterium that causes puerperal fever. In Meigs's defense, it should be noted that Pasteur's proof did not emerge until twenty-five years later. He was, moreover, only one of many prominent physicians who discounted the idea. Nevertheless, critics have held Meigs culpable, implying that Meigs was a reactionary whose intransigence prolonged the suffering of women for decades.[5]

Meigs's opposition to the use of obstetric anesthesia contributed to his reputation today as an insensitive reactionary. In his own time, however, he was in good company. Virtually the entire panoply of influential obstetricians sided with Meigs: Montgomery and Collins of Dublin, Ramsbotham and Tyler-Smith of London, Dubois of Paris, Scanzoni of Germany, Byford of Chicago, and Hodge of Philadelphia. A letter written by Robert Collins to Meigs illustrates the skepticism of most physicians: "I cordially agree in your observations on the use of chloroform. It is very little used either in Dublin or London by those whose practical experience entitles them to the confidence of their professional brethren." This comment flatly contradicts one made by Simpson: that Irish obstetricians were using anesthesia extensively. As late as 1856, Meigs wrote, "In Philadelphia, the use of ether and chloroform in surgery and midwifery has made no great progress, notwithstanding the very numerous reports upon the benefits derived from those agents in Europe." If true, this may reflect Meigs's strong influence on his Philadelphia colleagues, for almost everywhere else the controversy had already subsided.[6]

The experience of two famous patients exemplifies the reluctance of the medical profession to accept obstetric anesthesia. The first involved Fanny Appleton Longfellow, wife of the poet Henry Wadsworth Longfellow and the first woman in the United States to be anesthetized for childbirth. Apparently, Fanny and Henry kept abreast of medical innovations, seeking out and trying any that caught their attention. The Longfellows learned of obstetric anesthesia soon after Simpson's original announcement and resolved to try it during Fanny's impending confinement. Unable to find a Boston physician willing to administer ether, Fanny sought help from a dentist, Nathan Cooley Keep. At that time dentists were actively investigating the anesthetic properties of ether and probably used it more often than physicians. With Keep's help, Fanny gave birth in April 1847, barely four months after Simpson first used anesthesia in Edinburgh. All went well. Fanny wrote glowing comments about anesthesia to her friends and family, commenting that their fear for her safety had been unwarranted. She also chided Boston physicians for their "timidity." Keep, the man who anesthetized her, later became dean of the dental school at Harvard.[7]

The second famous patient, the queen of England, had three deliveries in the 1850s. Many aristocratic English women had been using anesthesia for childbirth when Sir Charles Locock, accoucheur to Queen Victoria, consulted

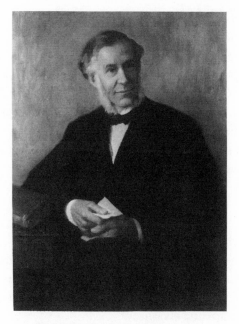

Nathan Cooley Keep (1800–1875).
Courtesy of the Harvard Medical Library
in the Francis A. Countway Library
of Medicine, Boston.

John Snow—a London physician already known for his skill
with anesthesia—about anesthetizing the queen for her confinement in 1850. Locock declined to use anesthesia for that
particular delivery, but he did ask Snow to anesthetize Victoria for her next delivery, three years later. Victoria's physicians made no public announcement of their use of anesthesia, but the news surfaced anyway, prompting the irascible
Thomas Wakley, founding editor of the medical journal the

Lancet, to write a scathing editorial. In it he criticized the queen's physicians for risking her life by using a dangerous drug simply to relieve the pain of labor. Neither the queen nor her physicians commented publicly, which was perhaps a prudent response to a strong attack from an influential physician. In 1857 Locock again asked Snow to anesthetize Victoria for her ninth and last delivery. This time there was no furor and no editorial, for the use of obstetric anesthesia had ceased to be a controversial medical issue.[8]

The Case Against Anesthesia

Debate about anesthesia was not restricted to obstetrics. During the early days of anesthesia, a similar argument developed around its use in surgery. The use of anesthesia forced physicians to develop new ways to weigh the risks and benefits of therapeutic measures.[9]

Many physicians thought the risks of anesthesia too high and, therefore, resisted its use. Nicolai Pirogoff, an eminent Russian surgeon, wrote: "To a surgeon steeled by courage, judgement, and experience to disagreeable and unwelcome screams and reactions to pain of his patients, an operation performed on a person robbed of feeling and consciousness is bound to be repugnant." Harsh as his words sound, he simply meant that surgeons relied on the reactions of their awake patients to guide surgery. Masking such reactions with anesthesia, he feared, would expose patients to greater risks. Pirogoff made similar remarks about anesthesia and obstetrics: "And, finally, haven't midwives and parturients and indeed all others always viewed the agonies of delivery as an indicator of safety and a well-nigh holy accompaniment of childbirth?" Remarkably, Pirogoff later overcame "those scruples . . . and became convinced that ether vapor is incontestably a remedy worthy of close attention." He even performed early studies of ether and wrote one of the first textbooks on anesthesia.[10]

In the mid-nineteenth century, risk-benefit ratios were easier to establish for surgery than for obstetrics. Patients submitted to surgery only if they were already close to death. Birthing, as conservative physicians observed, was quite different. Childbirth was said to be "natural," a process that "a kindly providence has so ordered . . . that the accoucheur, in most cases hath really nothing to do except to receive and protect the child and attend to the delivery of the afterbirth." Over and over, experts admonished midwives and practitioners to "remember the oft repeated adage, 'a meddlesome midwifery is bad,' and be therefore willing to abstain from impertinent interference." At that time, "impertinent interference" included the use of ergot, forceps, and other mechanical maneuvers to hasten the delivery. The risks of childbirth were too small to justify using anesthesia, it was thought. Meigs, not Simpson, spoke for most obstetricians.[11]

Simpson did not deny that anesthesia entailed risk. He did, however, attack the premise that pain is a normal part of childbirth. He said that regardless of the issue of survival for both mother and child, the pain of childbirth is destructive in and of itself, and this fact alone justified using anesthesia. Simpson not only contradicted traditional teaching but elevated the debate about pain to a new level.

Meigs and his allies examined Simpson's arguments and discovered several weak points. They rejected his attempt to equate surgical pain with obstetric pain. Critics also rejected Simpson's thesis that all pain is unnatural and destructive and must therefore be treated. The influential London obstetrician William Tyler-Smith spoke of the "manifold wisdom with which the act of parturition is surrounded"; the nature and severity of the pain, he said, did not justify incurring risks associated with anesthesia. Meigs and others called the routine use of anesthesia for labor pain a dangerous and "meddling" form of obstetric practice. Tyler-Smith wrote that "women will derive truer comfort and a greater measure of safety and freedom from unnecessary suffering from physiology, than from wild therapeutics, which in her hour of trial only offer a choice betwixt poison and pain."[12]

Identifying the specific risks of anesthesia proved difficult. It was known that anesthesia could kill; the first reports of fatalities had appeared within a very short time. That none of these deaths had involved obstetric patients prompted advocates of anesthesia to speculate that pregnancy was somehow protective. Needless to say, not everyone was mollified by this argument.[13]

Opponents of obstetric anesthesia raised another substantive issue when they suggested that anesthesia might adversely affect the birth process. Anesthesia might diminish uterine contractions, for example, or interfere with the well-being of the newborn child. Although opponents acknowledged that such problems were not lethal, the difficulties seemed sufficient to warrant limiting the use of the drug. Such reservations reflect uncertainty about the physiologic relation between uterine pain and uterine contractions. Meigs and most others discounted Simpson's comment that the two events were distinct and unrelated. They cited instances in which contractions had diminished during administration of anesthesia, and wondered how others could fail to notice such a response (years later their observations were substantiated). Opponents of anesthesia also pointed with derision to inconsistencies in the arguments of advocates such as Walter Channing, who had recommended that anesthesia be used to diminish "overly strong" contractions while at the same time declaring that ether and chloroform did not produce such effects.

Meigs and his allies criticized the rhetoric and tactics used by advocates of anesthesia, not just their facts and logic. In a vitriolic attack in the *Lancet*, the London obstetrician Robert Barnes aimed a sharp barb at Simpson: "When I asked what warranted Dr. Simpson in using so powerful an agent in natural labour, I was triumphantly answered that the professor had tried it on himself! I might object that the professor was not in labour, and that this was another instance of false analogy. The eleven cases of chloroformization Dr. Simpson detailed in his original proclamation, I did not think of a nature to justify his encomiums." [14] Similar charges were leveled against the encomiums generated by other advocates of anesthesia. From Paris, F. W. Fischer wrote how "a kind of insane ethereal furor had taken possession of the French Medical Mind for the purpose of testing its [ether's] powers." Tyler-Smith wrote how "a year ago . . . all women were promised safe and perfect exemption from the pains of natural labor" in the "most glowing and hyperbolic praises of the virtues of this intoxicating agent." He believed it only a matter of time before the "anaesthetic Elixir proves to be but a cup of Circe." Meigs dismissed Simpson's exaggerated claims with disdain: "In speaking of the various points in the conduct of a labor, I cannot well eschew to say something upon the employment of those anesthetic agents whose recent irruption into the domain of Medicine and Surgery has been so sudden, violent, and overbearing. To avoid altogether any notice of these agents would have been more consistent with my taste as well as my views of medical duty." [15]

Physicians complained that the publicity surrounding the introduction of obstetric anesthesia made it virtually impossible to obtain accurate information, particularly about problems. Francis Ramsbotham called it an "uphill fight" and wrote that "favorable cases are blazoned abroad with all the eagerness inspired by novelty and with all the éclat attendant on presumed success; whilst those in which any casualties have occurred are, for the most part, kept back from the eye of the public." Barnes noted how reports about "sundry ominous mishaps" slowly "ooze out, now and then." [16]

Another London physician decried Simpson's direct appeal to the public: "I did not expect that Dr. Simpson would have appealed so directly, and through so many channels, to the feelings and imperfect knowledge of society in general, for it is, I am happy to say, still very uncommon, in our profession, to find those of its members who would give tone to its bearing and conduct, professors, for instance, of our ancient universities, going about from one city to another to announce and exhibit the wonder effects of a new gas, and, as I am informed, somewhat after the fashion of a showman, to demonstrate them personally, at dinner parties, and in drawing rooms." [17]

Walter Channing, a Lone Source of Support

As a prototype of medical hyperbole and obfuscation, the critics of anesthesia might have cited *A Treatise on Etherization in Childbirth, Illustrated by Five Hundred Eighty-One Cases.* [18] Its author was Walter Channing (1786–1876), obstetrician and dean of Harvard Medical School. In the first

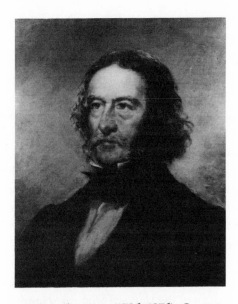

Walter Channing (1786–1876). Courtesy
of the Harvard Medical Library in the
Francis A. Countway Library of
Medicine, Boston.

years of obstetric anesthesia he was Simpson's only significant medical ally.

In influence and professional stature, Channing was
equal to Meigs and Simpson. Channing was one of three sons
of a prominent Rhode Island family. One brother, Edward,
became a professor of rhetoric at Harvard; another brother,
William, became a well-known cleric who rebelled against
the conservative Calvinistic doctrines of New England con-
gregational churches and helped to establish Unitarianism as
a separate denomination. Both Edward and William taught
and influenced such New England notables as Ralph Waldo

Emerson and Henry David Thoreau and thus helped shape the early Transcendental movement.

Walter Channing was expelled from Harvard when he was a junior for participating in the Bread and Butter Riot of 1805, so he moved to Philadelphia to study medicine at the University of Pennsylvania. After graduation, he continued medical studies in Edinburgh, a common pattern among ambitious young American graduates who wanted to gain more experience and polish before entering practice. Returning to Boston, he joined the Harvard faculty. In 1815 he became a lecturer on obstetrics and medical jurisprudence, joining Jacob Bigelow and John C. Warren, two physicians who were to play an important role in William Morton's demonstration of the first successful use of surgical anesthesia in 1846. In 1818 Channing was promoted to professor and only one year later became dean of the Harvard Medical School. Channing may be the only undergraduate in the history of American medicine who was expelled from a prestigious university only to return a few years later to become one of its deans. Channing was dean when Oliver Wendell Holmes moved from Dartmouth College to join the faculty of Harvard Medical School.[19]

Channing, like Simpson, called the "remedy of pain [a] noble subject." Like Simpson, he acknowledged that the effects of anesthesia on mother and child should be the major issue governing the use of ether. He hoped that his book would "contribute something towards settling the most important point concerning its further use, namely that of its safety."[20]

Channing chose an unusual way to settle issues of safety: a survey. By letter, he solicited opinions about anesthesia from those who had used it. He even asked Meigs, an action that says more about his courage than about his wisdom. He collated the replies and tempered them with his own experience to arrive at a consensus. The resulting book gave obstetric anesthesia a glowing recommendation.

Channing's approach had three faults. First, he included only the observations of patients given anesthesia. He left others the task of collecting comparative statistics—that is, descriptions of deliveries without anesthesia. Today such an effort would be discounted for its lack of appropriate controls. Second, he claimed that he had omitted descriptions of "untoward" results because none had been reported to him. In fact, several untoward results were mentioned in the book but were attributed to factors other than the anesthetic. Third, he presented many contradictions that conservative physicians found objectionable. Within the space of a few pages, Channing said that experience had taught him that ether might increase contractions, decrease contractions, and have no effect at all. He dismissed this conundrum by saying that "whatever ether's effect on the action of the uterus, it leads to a natural state of uterine function and consequently [he] welcomes it."

Some of Channing's suppositions even contradicted current medical knowledge. Channing claimed that ether given to the mother could not affect the child because it did not cross the placenta. He came to this conclusion because he could not detect the odor of ether at the cut ends of the umbilical cord. Although principles of physiology were poorly developed in 1848, this line of reasoning ran counter to existing knowledge about the transfer of materials across biologic membranes, including the placenta. Had he tried, Channing could have smelled ether on the exhalations of the newborn, as another physician did a short time later. The book's shortcomings notwithstanding, it had a tremendous impact on physicians and the public.[21]

Simpson, Meigs, and Channing had much in common despite their ideological differences. All three were products of a medical tradition shaped in Edinburgh. Simpson trained in Edinburgh and became one of its most famous graduates and professors. Channing studied in Edinburgh, and he and Meigs were graduates of the University of Pennsylvania, a school founded by Edinburgh graduates. Among the traditions transported from Edinburgh to Philadelphia was a high regard for instruction in obstetrics, a view unusual in medical education at that time.

The medicine taught at the University of Pennsylvania Medical School was highly influenced by William Cullen (1710–1790), one of Edinburgh's best-known medical educators. A dominant medical figure during the last decades of the eighteenth century, Cullen was famous as a clinician and as the author of an influential textbook. His reputation and teaching ability attracted many students from the colonies and from all over Europe. Americans who studied with Cullen included John Morgan, William Shippen, and Benjamin Rush, three of the original faculty of the University of Pennsylvania Medical School. It was Cullen's system of humoral medicine, of which more will be said later, that they brought to Philadelphia.[22]

Cullen's death in 1790 marked the end of an era in medicine. After his death, medicine changed quickly from a system following ancient Greek concepts to the scientific system that we know today. Coincident with the conversion in practice was a change in the expectations of patients. In effect, Simpson, Meigs, and Channing trained in one medical epoch and died in another. Conceptually and practically, the two epochs were separated by far more than a few decades. The responses of physicians to the challenge of anesthesia during the transition reflected their ties to both the old and the new forms of medicine. Of the three pioneers, Simpson may have been best prepared to cope with the new era.

"Bled, Leeched, Salivated"

The Transformation of Medical Practice by Science

I have been on the sick list repeatedly . . . with headaches

. . . and have been bled, leeched, salivated. I had a plateful

and a half of blood taken from me one night.

—James Young Simpson,

letter to his fiancée, Jessie Grindlay, 1836

J ust eleven years before James Young Simpson used ether to anesthetize a woman for delivery, he had used leeches, bleeding, and salivants to treat his own headache. This leap epitomized the change in medicine that occurred during the first half of the nineteenth century. When Charles Meigs and Walter Channing entered medical school in the first decade, the transition had not yet started. Even when Simpson enrolled in 1828, the change was barely under way. Yet within a few years medicine had evolved from a collection of folk remedies to the system of clinical science practiced today. Physicians had just begun to learn a new system of medicine when they found themselves also having to confront the mystery of anesthesia.

The greatest challenge of anesthesia was its potency. Chloroform and ether relieved pain better and faster than any existing herbal remedies. They abolished pain, but they also altered pulse rate, respiration, and other vital functions. Sometimes anesthesia killed with alarming speed. In 1846, the year of the Boston dentist William Morton's first successful demonstration of surgical anesthesia, physicians had no established methods for testing new drugs. Pharmacology was in its infancy. The anatomic and physiologic basis of modern medicine was just being developed. The transition from archaic to modern medicine coincided almost exactly with the careers of Simpson, Meigs, and Channing. By the time they all had died, the transition was virtually complete. Although they argued the merits of anesthesia, they had to cope with a much larger problem, an entirely new system of medical theory and practice. They used anesthesia before they were properly prepared to do so, and their reactions reflected their inexperience.[1]

Galenic Medicine

Simpson's choice of headache remedies typifies the archaic state of medicine early in the nineteenth century. For centuries physicians clung to ideas inherited from the ancient Greeks: that the body was composed of four elements— earth, air, fire, and water—each imbued with a primary quality, specifically, coldness, dryness, heat, or moisture. These elements combined in varying proportions to become the four "humors" of the body: blood, phlegm, yellow bile, and black bile. Like the elements that formed them, humors had distinctive characteristics and combined in various ways. A person's disposition reflected the mix of humors peculiar to his or her body. The temperament of one person might be "sanguine," reflecting an excessive amount of blood, "bilious," or "phlegmatic."[2]

According to Galen (circa 200 C.E.), the Greek physician most frequently credited with the advancement of humoral medicine, disease is a state in which the normal proportions of humors become unbalanced. To ascertain the nature of the imbalance, physicians observed a patient's disposition, then chose the therapy most likely to restore a normal balance. Techniques included bleeding, purging, and cupping (applying warm cups to the skin to raise blisters and draw out bad humors), and the use of cathartics, emetics, and salivants. For a disorder caused by an "excess of moisture," they might have prescribed an emetic or a cathartic.

Galen's system underwent considerable change during the millennium after his death—especially after the Renaissance, when physicians reexamined old manuscripts and found errors of fact and theory. In the 1550s Vesalius and Fabricius corrected Galen's anatomic descriptions, just as the English physician William Harvey (1578-1657) challenged his explanation of the circulation of blood. About the same time other physicians, such as Paracelsus (1493-1541) and Van Helmont (1577-1644), developed theories of body function and disease based on concepts of chemistry that were distinct from humoral theories derived from Galenic medicine. Somewhat later, Hermann Boerhaave (1668-1738) of Leiden and Friedrich Hoffman (1660-1742) of Halle discounted the theory of humors altogether and suggested that all disease came from a disruption of mechanical or physical forces. Almost simultaneously, Georg Stahl (1660-1734) and Albrecht von Haller (1708-1777) said that the nervous system regulated all bodily functions and that disease was simply a manifestation of some "nervous imbalance." Galenic medicine came to encompass humoral, mechanical, and neurologic theories of disease. Common to all these theories was the idea that disease is systemic, involving simultaneous dysfunction of all body parts. This justified the use of such systemic remedies as cupping, bleeding, and purging. The influence of Galenic theories peaked in Edinburgh during the last decades of the eighteenth century through the work of William Cullen (1710-1790).[3]

Cullen, one of Europe's most influential teachers, studied in Glasgow and taught there until 1766. When he moved to Edinburgh to join the medical faculty there, he took with him an outstanding reputation as a consultant, teacher, and author. Cullen died before Simpson, Meigs, or Channing began their careers, but his system of practice continued to dominate medical education, particularly in Edinburgh and Philadelphia.[4]

Cullen practiced a variant of Galenic medicine. Like Stahl and von Haller, he believed that disruptions of nervous "tension," or "excitement," were the cause of disease. A healthy body maintained a normal balance of excitatory and depressive stimuli. Disease suggested an imbalance. Excessive excitement increased muscle tone, disrupting circulation, digestion, and other bodily functions. A deficiency of nervous tension, on the other hand, might cause complete collapse. Cullen taught students to assess a patient's level of nervous excitement and then to adjust that level with either "stimulants," such as exercise, fresh air, warm wine, or tonic drugs, or with "depressants," such as rest, purging, bloodletting, or a meatless diet. When William Shippen, John Morgan, and Benjamin Rush established America's first medical school in Philadelphia, they used Cullen's variant of Galenic medicine as their model. Cullen's teaching thus linked Simpson, a graduate of Edinburgh, to Channing and Meigs, graduates of the University of Pennsylvania.[5]

Benjamin Rush modified Cullen's system and extended its influence in the United States and Europe. A native of Philadelphia, Rush apprenticed there with a local physician, moved to Edinburgh to obtain a medical degree, and traveled to London and Paris for informal study in other hospitals. His affability, intelligence, and an introductory letter from Benjamin Franklin smoothed his entry into exclusive medical and social circles. In Edinburgh he became close to his teacher William Cullen and to the Scottish philosopher David Hume. In London he worked with William Hunter, the famous surgeon and founder of the Hunterian School of Medicine, and dined with Samuel Johnson, the great lexicographer. When Rush returned to Philadelphia, he joined Morgan and Shippen on the faculty of the University of Pennsylvania and became one of the most influential teachers at the medical school, partly because of his medical work and partly because of his reputation as a patriot.[6]

Throughout his career Rush moved easily and often between medicine and politics. He served twice as a member of the Continental Congress, signed the Declaration of Independence, and became surgeon general of the Revolutionary Army. An early advocate for the humane treatment of the insane, he initiated a number of important social reforms. During the yellow fever epidemic of 1793, he risked his own life by staying in Philadelphia to organize and direct a cadre of medical workers to care for the ill and dying, an act that enhanced his already illustrious reputation. Upon learning of Rush's death, Thomas Jefferson wrote to John Adams, "Another of our friends of '76 is gone, my dear Sir, another of the co-signers of the independence of our country. And a better [man] than Rush, could not have left us more benevolent, more learned, of finer genius, or more honest."[7] One contemporary called Rush "America's Sydenham," an allusion to an illustrious early English physician. Undoubtedly, Rush's social, political, and medical prominence helped him to disseminate his ideas.

Although Rush retained Cullen's idea that the nervous system governs all body functions, he eliminated the concept of balance, a key feature of many early theories of disease. Rush believed that disease came from overstimulation, which caused "excessive motion of the arteries," by which he probably meant a rapid and bounding pulse. Because he ascribed all disease to overstimulation, he recommended only one kind of therapy: depressants. He was particularly fond of bloodletting and purging and used them aggressively. "Plethora," an excessive accumulation of blood, he noted, was part of every pregnancy—not an unreasonable statement in view of the edema and venous distention that normally occur. Rush said that this plethora caused excessive motion of the arteries, another normal change. Rush assumed, however, that a bounding rapid pulse necessarily signified a problem. To forestall complications, he advised physicians to counteract plethora by bleeding women often during pregnancy.[8]

Rush used bloodletting to treat other obstetric problems. He thought that excessive motion of the arteries caused by plethora overstimulated the brain, inducing the convulsions commonly associated with toxemia. To treat convulsions, he removed large amounts of blood while the patients were standing upright. Undoubtedly the ensuing shock stopped the convulsions or at least their outward manifestations. Rush claimed that bloodletting also hastened delivery and lessened labor pain.[9]

Presumably, the simplicity of these ideas was part of their appeal, for Rush's system became popular in Europe as well as the United States. Rush died in 1813, four years before Meigs finished medical school, but his influence continued for some time thereafter.

Though fanciful by today's standards, Rush's system resembled other styles of medical practice common during the nineteenth century. A few decades earlier, the Austrian physician Anton Mesmer developed a therapeutic system based on "animal magnetism." Animal magnetism, he claimed, would cure all types of medical problems. King Louis XVI thought this controversial theory important enough to warrant study by a special committee. Benjamin Franklin, then ambassador to France, chaired the committee, which was composed of five members of the Academy of Science. Not long afterward, Robert Thompson, an American, developed "botanic" medicine, and Samuel Hahnemann, a German, developed "homeopathy," which survives to this day. The last significant innovation of this sort may have been "Christian Scientism," the system of healing founded by Mary Baker Eddy in the middle of the nineteenth century.[10]

These four systems attribute all disease to systemic or

"humoral" factors. Accordingly, they emphasize systemic or "holistic" treatment. For these characteristics and for their aggressive use of unproven therapies they have been classified as forms of "heroic medicine." In an age when unfettered conjecture governed medical practice, Rush, however, reigned supreme. He is said to have single-handedly popularized the use of speculation among a whole generation of American medical graduates.[11]

Eventually, the therapeutic excesses of heroic medicine evoked a strong reaction. Physicians criticized the old systems and then discarded them. Small cracks began to appear in Rush's medical reputation even before he died. As early as 1793, one critic derided Rush's bleeding therapy for yellow fever as "one of those great medical discoveries which have helped to depopulate the earth." Within a generation his medical reputation was in tatters. In 1851 the physician and medical critic Elisha Barrett wrote of Rush's publications that "in the whole vast compass of medical literature, there cannot be found an equal number of pages containing a greater amount and variety of utter nonsense and unqualified absurdity." Seldom has one physician's reputation risen so high and fallen so far in so short a time.[12]

Cullen's influence also dwindled as his medical school lost stature. Several factors contributed to Edinburgh's decline. One was the disruption caused by continuous bickering among faculty members. Simpson himself fueled this problem through his lifelong feud with Syme, the surgeon who had opposed his appointment to the faculty. Another was the waning of the energy and originality of the Edinburgh faculty, as illustrated by the story of the three Monros. Alexander Monro (primus), a student of Boerhaave's, helped found the Edinburgh Medical School in 1726 and was its first professor of anatomy. His son, Monro secundus, succeeded him and also enjoyed an excellent reputation. The grandson, Monro tertius, had neither the flair nor the skill of his antecedents. He read his lectures verbatim from notes penned by his grandfather. Students, bored by his poor presentations, preferred to study anatomy with extra-academic teachers. Finally, just before Simpson's matriculation, the school lost more prestige because of the scandal of Burke and Hare, two criminals who murdered citizens of Edinburgh to sell their bodies for anatomical dissection. Outraged, mobs of citizens rioted and threatened the safety of some of the medical faculty, including Robert Knox, the extra-academic teacher whose lectures had stimulated Simpson to study medicine.[13]

Coincident with Edinburgh's decline was the growing reputation of French medicine. Liberated by the intellectual achievements of the Enlightenment and by the political consequences of the American and French Revolutions, French medical schools came to encourage independent thought, formerly an attribute only of Scottish schools, and they had additional advantages that had never existed in Scotland, such as a ready supply of inexpensive cadavers. Law and custom in France, unlike that in Scotland and England, permitted autopsies and encouraged human dissection. The importance of an abundant supply of cadavers should not be underestimated. Throughout the nineteenth century the study of anatomy occupied the same critical place in medical theory and education that is now filled by the field of molecular biology.[14] Essential knowledge gained through anatomical dissection was the basis for the revolution in the theory and practice of medicine.

French sensibilities also permitted animal experimentation. Accordingly, physiology flourished under the leadership of François Magendie and, later, Claude Bernard. In England, on the other hand, the rising spirit of humanism extended to animals. Even prominent physicians disparaged animal experimentation. Reluctance to experiment with animals retarded the development of any significant school of physiology in England until late in the nineteenth century, thereby impeding the development of English medicine.[15] For example, Magendie and the Scottish physician Charles Bell made the distinction between sensory and motor nerves almost simultaneously, yet Magendie received more credit because he supported his observations with animal experiments.

The French system of medicine that replaced the medical constructs of Cullen and Rush had three important attributes: close observation of the physical changes associated with disease; correlation of clinical signs and symptoms at the bedside with anatomic findings at the autopsy; and meticulous classification of disease by means of premortem and postmortem observations. This new system led physicians to a closer study of the structure and function of different tissues and organs. To enhance examination of the body, medical scientists used new tools and methods, such as the stethoscope (invented by Laënnec), the ophthalmoscope (Helmholtz), the microscope (Leuwenhoek), and percussion (Auenbrugger). In addition, they used mathematical methods to study disease, analyze data, and evaluate treatment. Credit for popularizing "numerical medicine" goes to the French physician Pierre Charles-Alexandre Louis (1787–1872), who published *Recherches sur les effét de la saignée* in 1835. Louis, a founder of medical statistics, had a major influence on the development of both French medicine and American medicine through the many students who worked with him. It was a form of "numerical analysis" that finally demonstrated the folly of aggressive bloodletting, for instance. Two American students of Louis, Henry Bigelow and

Oliver Wendell Holmes, were among the Harvard physicians who played a important role in Morton's first successful demonstration of anesthesia.[16]

Changes in medical thought and methods had several effects. As descriptions of diseases became more detailed and precise and as knowledge of body functions increased, physicians recognized the inadequacy of unitary explanations of disease, like those proposed by Cullen and Rush. Instead, physicians looked for causes unique to specific organs and tissues. The new system was critical of ungrounded theory. As the scientific movement matured, physicians discounted theories of any sort and relied solely on the empirical use of "observation" and "fact." They thought that given a collection of observations of high quality and sufficient number, the principles underlying natural phenomena would become evident without the need for a hypothesis. So great was their distrust of theory that empiricism itself was rejected once it was recognized to be a medical philosophy in its own right.[17]

Old and New Medical Theories in Obstetric Practice

Although Simpson, Meigs, and Channing trained at a time when the theories of Cullen and Rush still dominated medicine, all three had contact with the new French system. After Simpson graduated from medical school he toured hospitals in Paris, and throughout his career he entertained a stream of foreign physicians at his Edinburgh home. Meigs had similar opportunities. He translated French obstetric textbooks into English, and many of his colleagues and contemporaries had studied in Paris because of the shift in political alignments after the wars of 1776 and 1812 and because the excitement of French medicine had diverted American students from Edinburgh to Paris. Two of these students, William Wood

Gerhard and Samuel B. Gross, were contemporaries of Meigs who returned from Paris to establish distinguished careers in Philadelphia as teachers and writers. The situation in Boston was similar. Channing appointed George B. Shattuck and Oliver Wendell Holmes to the Harvard faculty; both had studied in Paris and had been particular favorites of their teacher Pierre Louis, a founder of medical statistics. Presumably they discussed the new French medical system with students and other faculty members. At the same time, American medical journals, many of them founded then, brought news of medical developments in France to Boston, New York, and Philadelphia and disseminated that news throughout the country.[18]

The obstetric practices of Meigs, Channing, and Simpson reflect their ties to both the old and the new forms of medicine. Their management of puerperal convulsions, a common obstetric problem, is illustrative.

When Meigs and Channing entered medical school, textbooks still attributed convulsions occurring during childbirth to plethora, as Rush and Cullen had. Plethora was thought to distend blood vessels of the uterus and the brain and to stimulate the nervous system, thereby causing convulsions. Predictably, standard textbooks recommended Rush's favorite treatments, bleeding and purging. Samuel Bard, a former student of Cullen's and cofounder of the second oldest medical school in America, King's College in New York City, wrote:

> Fits may probably be prevented by one or two moderate bleedings, by opening the bowels with salts and by keeping them free by occasional doses; by a low diet, cooling drinks, avoiding wine, much exercise and all violent passions. The same remedies are necessary after the fits have come on, only they must be applied with

greater vigour; the bleeding must be more copious, and if the blood be drawn from the jugular veins, or temporal artery, it will be most efficacious: at any rate, cupping glasses, with scarifications should be applied to the nape of the neck or temple; and the bleeding must be copious and repeated according to the violence of the symptoms and the strength of the patients.[19]

By 1873, about the time that Simpson and Meigs died, such theory and therapy had disappeared. William Leishman, professor of obstetrics at Glasgow, attributed convulsions of pregnancy to uremia, the accumulation of toxins in the body from kidney failure. For treatment he recommended administration of chloroform to stop the convulsions and to induce premature delivery of the child. Leishman's comments reflect the influence of French medicine. He spoke of chemical derangements, not a vague humoral imbalance like plethora, and attributed the underlying problem to failure of a specific organ, the kidney. Termination of pregnancy is a treatment still used today. Meigs's comments about the cause and management of puerperal convulsions are identical to those of Bard. Simpson, who trained a decade later, seems more ambivalent. In lecture notes he cites "excessive blood" as a cause of convulsions but suggests uremia and excess carbonate or chloride as other possibilities.[20] For treatment he mentions bleeding but questions its effectiveness. In this respect, Simpson seems closer to Leishman than to Bard.

Medical Theory and Anesthesia

The reactions of Simpson, Meigs, and Channing to anesthesia also reflect the old and the new styles of medicine. Simpson's ideas about labor pain resemble those of Rush and Cullen. Simpson believed labor pain could stimulate the nervous system, thereby causing convulsions or permanent damage. He differed from Rush only in his preference for anesthesia rather than bloodletting to suppress nervous tension, which was "otherwise liable to be produced by such pain," and thus gain an escape "from many evil consequences that are too apt to follow in its train."[21] Even though Simpson appears modern for recommending anesthesia, his reasons for doing so were decidedly not.

Simpson's style of presentation is reminiscent of an earlier era. Like Rush and Cullen, he relied on analogy, reason, and rhetoric rather than the methods of observation and analysis used by the French. He never offered data to support his contention that the pain of childbirth could damage or kill. Citing Galen's aphorism "Pain is useless to the pained" was another gaffe. French skepticism had discounted the opinions of such "authorities." Physicians who adopted the critical and analytic methods of French physicians had reason to complain about the encomiums, false analogies, and hyperbole used to promote obstetric anesthesia.

But Simpson's critics also relied on rhetoric. Although one of them, Meigs, argued that labor and its pain were "physiologic," he never defined the word nor offered experimental proof. His predilection for conjecture seemed excessive even to his contemporaries. In one review, a commentator criticized Meigs for his "affected obscure style and fondness for speculations, which, however brilliant and ingenious they may appear, are in many instances baseless as visions. . . . His fondness for what is speculative leads him often to prefer what is novel, ingenious and peculiarly his own, to that which is more worthy of and sanctioned by a common acception."[22] In this regard, Meigs's style, like Simpson's, resembles that which French physicians had discarded.

In contrast, Simpson and Channing appeared progressive when they suggested using numbers to evaluate obstetric anesthesia. Still, Channing only talked about statistics; he did not use them. Simpson did use statistics to demonstrate the benefits of anesthesia for leg amputations, which suggests he knew something of the work of Louis. Simpson would have been more credible had he also used numbers to demonstrate the benefits of anesthesia for childbirth. Meigs's attitude toward statistics, on the other hand, was reactionary. He never acknowledged their value for any medical problem, much less for obstetric anesthesia—nor did his contemporary Claude Bernard, one of the world's first great experimental physiologists.[23]

In spite of Meigs's recalcitrance regarding statistics, he appeared modern when he called obstetric anesthesia "meddlesome." French physicians stressed the healing power of nature. The body would maintain itself quite well, they said, if left alone. Physicians should not interfere; they should use only those remedies that promote natural processes. Meigs's opposition to anesthesia fell in line with ongoing controversies about other "meddlesome" practices, such as the use of ergots and forceps. He knew that anesthesia stopped labor pain but maintained that the pain was inextricably bound to labor. Meigs's strong reaction may reflect his antipathy toward the residual influence of his fellow Philadelphian Benjamin Rush, whose name had become synonymous with meddlesome, dangerous, and irrational medical practices.

Physicians involved in the early debates about obstetric anesthesia recognized its potential and its risks. Channing, for one, undertook to learn whether anesthesia was "safe both to mother and to child." Simpson went one step further when he identified the different components of the problem: the effects of anesthesia on labor, on the child, and on mortality. Virtually all the work done since 1847 has focused on issues that Simpson originally identified. As it turned out, resolving the problems was far more difficult than anyone could have imagined. Physicians were not prepared to deal with such complex issues. They knew little about the normal physiology of the uterus, much less about its response to drugs. They had only the barest insight into placental function, much less about the permeability of the placenta to ether and chloroform. They knew nothing about the physiologic adaptation of the neonate to extrauterine life, much less about how drugs might affect these processes. They knew nothing about the mechanisms that control postpartum hemorrhage, much less about factors that alter the risk of postpartum infection. Most important, they had no experience in research methods, including statistical analysis. Medicine was just emerging from its own dark age.

Even had Simpson, Meigs, and Channing the inclination to take up such problems, it is doubtful that they would have had the time. All had hectic careers as clinicians, educators, and writers. Simpson often slept on the floor of railway cars as he returned to Edinburgh after examining patients in nearby cities. Meigs and Channing had one more handicap, living as they did in America during the "Age of Jackson"—public sentiment favored technical innovation, not science. The public had little interest in supporting work that had no immediate or demonstrable benefit. This was a handicap, because many clinical questions pertaining to obstetric anesthesia could not be answered until scientists acquired knowledge about underlying physiologic mechanisms. Such information was forthcoming, but not for almost half a century, and then from a group of physicians working at an entirely different location.

"The Queen in Her Confinement"

John Snow's Approach to Anesthesia

Administered chloroform to the Queen in her confinement.

Slight pains had been experienced since Sunday. Dr. Locock was

sent for about nine o'clock this morning, stronger pains having

commenced, and he found the os uteri had commenced to

dilate a very little. I received a note from Sir James Clark a

little after ten asking me to go to the Palace. I remained in

an apartment near that of the Queen, along with Sir J. Clark,

Dr. Ferguson and Dr. Locock till a little a[fter] twelve. At twenty

minutes past twelve by a clock in the Queen's apartment

I commenced to give a little chloroform with each pain,

by pouring about 15 minims by measure on a folded handkerchief. The first stage of labour was nearly over when the chloroform was commenced. Her Majesty expressed great relief from the application, the pains being very trifling during the uterine contractions, and whilst between the periods of contraction there was complete ease. The chloroform was not at any time carried to the extent of quite removing consciousness. . . . The infant was born at 13 minutes past one by the clock in the room; consequently the chloroform was inhaled for 53 minutes. The placenta was expelled in a very few minutes, and the Queen appeared very cheerful and well, expressing herself much gratified with the effect of the chloroform.

—*The Case Books of Dr. John Snow,* 1848–1857

Applying new medical methods to obstetric care took more time and effort than Simpson, Meigs, and Channing might have imagined. Identifying problems associated with anesthesia was simple. Solving them was not. Few people had the ability or the interest to persevere. A notable exception was John Snow, a London physician.[1]

To many, Snow personified the ideal nineteenth-century physician. He was observant, thoughtful, inquisitive, and critical. Most important, he was a clinician and, by all accounts, a very good one. To explore the medical effects of ether and chloroform, he also became an investigator, using discoveries about chemical and physical principles that were just emerging from European laboratories to solve clinical problems. Even by today's standards, Snow's work is exemplary for its simplicity, originality, and accuracy. In short, he possessed traits that modern medical schools try to inculcate in all their graduates. Remarkably, Snow appears to have determined his methods on his own. His formal education was modest, and he had no special training in science or research, nor had he direct contact with the medical tradition developing in French hospitals.

Snow had a keen interest in applying anesthesia to obstetrics. He anesthetized many women of the English aristocracy for childbirth. The technique was entirely his own and became the method favored by obstetricians for almost a century. In style, substance, and lasting influence, Snow stands in sharp contrast to Simpson, Meigs, and Channing.

Snow, the Queen's Anesthetist

Born in 1813, the year Benjamin Rush died, Snow was practicing medicine in London in 1846 when the dentist James

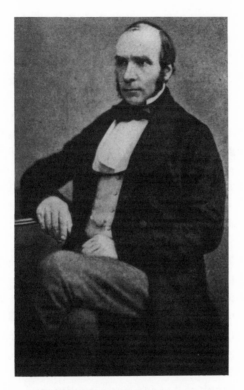

John Snow (1813–1858). Courtesy
of the Wood Library-Museum of
Anesthesiology, Chicago.

Robinson administered the first modern anesthetic in that
city. Fascinated by early reports, Snow gradually gave up
family practice in favor of anesthesia. Known for his competence, Snow became the favorite anesthetist for many of
London's foremost surgeons, including Robert Liston, from
whom Simpson had first learned about anesthesia.

Snow published two books on anesthesia. The first, a

slim volume entitled *On the Inhalation of the Vapour of Ether in Surgical Operations*, appeared in 1847. The second, a far more extensive book entitled *On Chloroform and Other Anaesthetics: Their Action and Administration*, was published shortly after his death in 1858. For every anesthetic that he gave, Snow kept detailed records including the name, age, and physical condition of the patient, the name of the surgeon, and details of the surgical procedure. These "case books" also included records of more than eighty-five anesthetics given for obstetric patients. It was Snow whom Queen Victoria's accoucheurs consulted during her confinement in 1850, and it was he whom they asked to administer anesthesia for her deliveries in 1853 and 1857.[2]

Snow's interest in science preceded his involvement with anesthesia. As long as he lived in London, he was active in the Westminster Medical Society, a private club that met regularly for medical presentations and discussion. Snow once served as the society's president and often gave lectures and demonstrations. His first presentation, "On Asphyxia, and On the Resuscitation of Stillborn Children," dealt with an obstetric problem. Subsequently published in the *London Medical Gazette*, it covered intrauterine asphyxia, physiologic mechanisms responsible for the newborn's first breath, and ventilation of the apneic child by means of a special apparatus that Snow had built.[3]

Snow's flair for investigation also surfaced in epidemiology. Intrigued by the geographical distribution of cholera cases during an epidemic, he attributed the outbreak to contaminated water in one section of London. In spite of criticism from medical authorities, he persisted with his idea and eventually prevailed. His work, the first demonstration of a water-borne disease, helped to initiate development of public health measures to ensure the purity of drinking water.

Remarkably, Snow's investigation preceded by several years both the discovery of bacteria and the announcement of the germ theory of disease. For his work on cholera, Snow is universally recognized as one of the founders of epidemiology.[4]

In many respects, Snow's studies on anesthesia were also prescient. Safety was an important impetus for his work. Soon after the introduction of chloroform, reports appeared of unexpected deaths, some of which occurred after patients had taken no more than one or two breaths of anesthetic. In several papers and in his last book, Snow analyzed the circumstances of these deaths and speculated about their cause. He knew that an overdose of anesthetic could kill. He also recognized that the clinical response to anesthesia varied with the dose administered. Snow attributed deaths and other mishaps to inadvertent overdoses of anesthetic caused by imprecise methods of administration, and concluded that physicians must learn to control the dose of anesthetic gases "to determine when it [anesthesia] had been carried far enough."[5]

Even today, estimating anesthetic dose can be a formidable task, but in 1847 it was particularly so. Having relied on poultices and herbs, nineteenth-century physicians had little experience with potent drugs. Of those drugs available to them—opium, digitalis leaf, calomel, quinine—few worked as fast or as effectively as anesthetics. Pharmacology, the study of the interaction between chemicals and the body, was in its infancy. Books on medicinal chemistry dealt more with the particulars of compounding prescriptions than with the details of drug action. Concepts dealing with, say, the relation between the dose of a drug and the response of the patient were only then being developed, and they remained unknown except to a handful of curious, better-informed physicians. Nor were there established methods to guide the study of the efficacy or side effects of new drugs, or agencies to evaluate the claims of manufacturers and medical entrepreneurs. To establish the pharmacologic properties of anesthetics, Snow had to find his own way.[6]

Snow divided the problem of anesthetic dose into two parts. First, he determined the sequence of bodily changes that occurred with the induction of anesthesia: altered consciousness, spontaneous movements, vocalization, reflex response to pain, and decreases in respiration and heart rate, among others. He used these events to estimate different degrees of anesthesia. Two famous French physiologists, Pierre Flourens and Claude Bernard, had done similar work, showing that various body functions tended to disappear in a particular sequence. Snow, however, found that each function also disappeared at a particular depth of anesthesia. Consciousness seemed to be most susceptible, disappearing first and after only a very small dose. Normal respiration and heart rate persisted much longer. Snow established the predictability of this sequence among humans and even among other species.

Snow also recognized several characteristics of the patient that could alter the response to anesthesia. He observed that the effect of a given dose varied with the patient's age, gender, any preexisting "hysteria," general physical condition, and even "level of education." He noticed that anesthetic requirements varied with severity of the pain and suggested that dosage be adjusted for the particular type of surgery. To him, an anesthetic "had been carried far enough" at the point of the best possible balance among all these variables. The principle was sound, and it guides anesthesia practice to this day.[7]

Having established a method to estimate different levels of anesthesia and having identified factors that may cause the level to vary, Snow sought to learn the amount of anesthetic vapor that would produce each level. This project required considerable ingenuity, for measuring the amount of gas to be inhaled was far more difficult than weighing the amount of a powder to be swallowed or liquid to be injected. Snow solved this problem by using what he had learned about the physical and chemical properties of ether and chloroform. Though liquids at room temperature, chloroform and ether vaporize quickly when placed in open containers. Snow used this property to make gas mixtures of known concentration. He put a measured volume of each liquid anesthetic into a bag of known capacity. He calculated the final concentration of the vaporized anesthetic, knowing that it varied in direct proportion to the original volume of liquid. He then exposed mice, guinea pigs, rabbits, birds, frogs, and an occasional cat to anesthetic mixtures of varying concentrations. By observing the response of the animals, he ascertained the amount (or concentration) that would kill and the amount that would induce the clinical signs that he had associated with different degrees, or levels, of anesthesia.

Snow's experiments suggest a thorough understanding of the gas laws, the principles that govern the behavior of gases in different physical conditions. He had an outstanding facility in using such information to solve clinical problems. He calculated the solubility of anesthetics in blood and the physical capacity of blood to absorb anesthetic vapors, and he speculated that the potency of an anesthetic was related to solubility, thereby anticipating by fifty years experiments on the mechanism of action of anesthetic gases.[8]

Realizing that temperature alters the rate of vaporization of ether and chloroform, Snow evaluated how temperature affected the solubility of anesthetic gases. He suspected, correctly, that uncontrolled changes in ambient temperature cause unexpected changes in the amount of anesthetic given to the patient: in a warm room the liquid anesthetic turns more easily into a vapor. To minimize fluctuations in the ambient temperature, he designed a special device to vaporize liquid anesthetics into a gas, a device that he used for much of his clinical work.

Though crude by today's standards, his device was vastly superior to other techniques then in use. Most physicians placed a piece of cloth over a patient's nose or mouth and poured liquid anesthetic onto the cloth until conditions were considered right for surgery. Snow spoke disparagingly of this method:

> According to Professor Miller, chloroform was given, at one time, in the Royal Infirmary of Edinburgh, in a somewhat slovenly, and not very cleanly manner; he describes the means of applying it as, "anything that will admit of chloroform in vapour being brought fully in contact with the mouth and nostrils; a handkerchief, a towel, a piece of lint, a worsted glove, a nightcap, a sponge." He says, "In the winter season, the glove of a clerk, dresser, or onlooker, has been not unfrequently pressed into the service. . . . The object is to produce insensibility as completely and so soon as we can; and there is no saying, a priori, whether this is to be accomplished by fifty drops or five hundred."[9]

With justification, Snow said that his method was better. For the more than eight hundred applications of anesthetics listed in his case books, he mentions only three anesthetic fatalities, a low death rate that was a remarkable achievement considering the serious condition of many of his patients and the complexity of some of the operations.

Snow and Obstetric Anesthesia

Snow used the same approach for obstetric anesthesia that he had used for surgical anesthesia. First, he defined the need for pain relief. He noted, for example, that women in labor often required a smaller dose of anesthetic but that they varied in their response. The dose administered, therefore, should also vary. Parturients who coped well might need none, he said, but those with great pain or little tolerance should be given more. For normal labors, Snow sought to abolish consciousness without suspending other body functions. So lightly were his patients anesthetized that most of them responded to commands and pushed appropriately during delivery of the child, even though they had little or no memory of labor pain. Because he used this method to anesthetize Queen Victoria, others labeled it *anesthesia à la Reine*.[10]

Having established a level of anesthesia appropriate for most obstetric patients, Snow described how to achieve it. To minimize exposure, he delayed starting the anesthetic until the patient was far advanced in labor, usually within an hour or two of delivery. He recommended giving only the smallest amount of anesthetic needed to relieve pain and then only during contractions while the patient actually felt pain. He suggested that the dose could be tapered down during labor because the anesthetic tends to accumulate in the body over time. In view of the increased susceptibility to anesthesia during pregnancy, the lengthiness of labor, and the variation in response among women, Snow thought it particularly important to control doses for obstetric patients carefully. He advised always using a vaporizer to ensure the most precise control over the inhaled concentrations of gas.[11]

Snow recognized several obstetric situations likely to increase the need for anesthesia, such as prolonged labor or malposition of the child. He also understood that anesthesia could be used for purposes other than the relief of pain. Accepting the fact that anesthesia could stop uterine contractions, he suggested some situations where this response might be useful—when relaxation of the uterus was needed to turn the child or for extraction of the afterbirth. Snow knew that contractions would return quickly once the anesthetic was discontinued and that the temporary diminution of contractions would not increase the risk of postpartum hemorrhage. Here, Snow differed from Channing and other early advocates of anesthesia who dismissed the possibility of uterine effects. He also differed from Meigs, who used the putative effects of anesthesia on the uterus as a reason to avoid using anesthesia altogether.[12]

Snow disliked Simpson's methods. Simpson started anesthesia early in labor, gave a lot of anesthesia, and made no attempt to tailor his technique to the needs of individual patients. He simply poured chloroform on a cloth placed over the patient's nose until she was unconscious and unresponsive, virtually the same technique that others used for surgery. However appropriate for amputations or extractions of bladder stones, procedures that last only a few minutes, this method was not appropriate for labor, which might last for hours. Snow said so and criticized Simpson's influence on others: "The high position of Dr. Simpson and his previous services in this department, more particularly in being the first to administer ether in labour, gave his recommendations very great influence; the consequence of which is, that the practice of anesthesia is presently probably in a much less satisfactory state than it would have been if chloroform had never been introduced."[13] Snow's comment is telling, considering that it came not from a critic of obstetric anesthesia but from one of its most articulate and effective proponents.

Snow's Early Life and Training

Given Snow's modest personal background, it is surprising that he accomplished so much. He was the eldest of nine children, his father a Yorkshire laborer. Snow and several siblings overcame this social and economic handicap to become successful in medicine, trade, the church, and education.

Snow's medical background was equally inauspicious. At age fourteen he began a five-year apprenticeship with a medical practitioner in Newcastle upon Tyne. After this, he served a second, shorter apprenticeship in Burnop Field, then worked for a year and a half as an assistant in a nearby hospital. He moved to London, where he enrolled in the Hunterian School of Medicine in 1836. Following a year of lectures, he "walked the wards" at nearby hospitals, the accepted method used by students to obtain clinical experience. In 1838 Snow was licensed by both the Royal College of Surgeons and the Society of Apothecaries. Although licensure by either organization qualified Snow to practice, neither conferred much social or professional prestige. Those who received an apothecary license were usually rural practitioners who treated those ailments likely to respond to herbs or drugs. Surgeons, who were just breaking free from the stigma of their long professional association with barbers, handled all other problems. Licentiates of both groups, apothocaries and surgeons, ranked lower than physicians, who had received their medical degree from a medical school or university. Snow aspired to become a physician.[14]

Eventually, Snow enrolled at the University of London,

the school founded by the political philosopher Jeremy Bentham and wealthy London Quakers and Methodists who wanted to provide a university education to those who could not satisfy the religious requirements for admission to Oxford or Cambridge. At the University of London, Snow qualified for two degrees: a bachelor's degree and a doctorate in medicine. With these credentials, he joined the next higher professional tier in English medicine. Still not satisfied, Snow sat for the examination to become a licentiate of the Royal College of Physicians. He passed, thus becoming a member of the highest professional stratum of physicians in nineteenth-century England.

Snow's medical training alone could not have prepared him for his work on the physical and chemical properties of medicinal gases. The Hunterian School of Medicine was founded during the eighteenth century by William Hunter, his brother John, and several colleagues, many of whom had studied with William Cullen in Glasgow before he moved to Edinburgh. Once it had ranked among the most prestigious private medical institutions in England, but its reputation and influence had diminished with each succeeding generation. Shortly after Snow finished his studies the school closed. There were several reasons for its demise: it could not compete with the hospital-based medical schools springing up in provincial cities, Oxford and Cambridge had improved their medical curricula, and large numbers of the English preferred to study medicine in France.[15]

Snow is more likely to have learned about the physical properties of gases from books or scientific papers than from lectures at school. By 1840 much was known about gases through the work of such early scientists as Robert Boyle (1627–1691), Joseph Louis Gay-Lussac (1778–1850), William Henry (1774–1836), John C. Dalton (1766–1844), and Robert

Wilhelm Bunsen (1811–1899). Several years earlier, the English physician Thomas Beddoes had aroused considerable public interest for his work at the Pneumatic Institute, a private clinic in Bristol where he explored therapeutic applications of several recently discovered gases, among them oxygen, carbon dioxide, nitrogen, and nitrous oxide. Sir Humphry Davy and Henry Hill Hickman, a protégé of Beddoes, carried this work further. Hickman had written a popular tract describing his work with nitrous oxide. Considering Snow's curiosity and work habits, he probably knew of these people and their work. We can only guess, however, for his books and papers contain no suggestion of a link, nor does his biography, written by Benjamin Ward Richardson, a physician and close friend.[16]

Snow and Simpson had much in common. Both were influential, highly respected Victorian physicians who made major contributions to medicine and to the management of obstetric pain. Born a few years and a few hundred miles apart, each came from a large, poor family. Each began medical studies at age fourteen. By virtue of Scottish support for education, Simpson studied at one of Europe's most prestigious medical schools. Snow, in contrast, started as an apprentice to a rural physician, but by his own effort and intellect acquired an exceptional education. But the two men with so much in common developed very different styles.

Bold, charismatic, and sometimes abrasive, Simpson had many characteristics of physicians in the previous century. He was flamboyant and, to the dismay of his colleagues, often appealed directly to the public.[17] Although they were somewhat influenced by the new French medical style, Simpson's practice retained many features of Galenic medicine. Fond of innovation and oblivious to impediments, Simpson used anesthesia like a broadsword. His approach to obstetric pain was devoid of nuance or subtlety and appears naive, even in the context of his own times.

In contrast, Snow's cautious, analytic, and critical style seems more consonant with modern medicine. He filled his notes, papers, and books with clinical observations but omitted speculation. Not satisfied with identifying problems, Snow sought to solve them. In doing so, he used many new principles and techniques from physics and chemistry and, in the process, developed clinical devices and techniques that appealed to his colleagues and survived for several decades.

After Snow, obstetric anesthesia changed. Clinicians who had originally opposed it began to use anesthesia cautiously. Some who had been outspoken critics of Simpson for advocating its use came to praise him instead. William Tyler-Smith, dedicating the 1858 edition of his textbook to Simpson, commented that "few would willingly enter upon general practice without the use of anaesthetics of some kind. . . . Any person sufficiently educated in medicine to take charge of a case of labor will have learnt the proper method of administration." Francis Ramsbotham, another early critic, dedicated the fifth edition of his textbook to Simpson, "whose indefatigable exertions in the cause of Science and successful efforts to alleviate human suffering have rendered his name famous throughout the world." Ramsbotham went on to admit that his early fear of obstetric anesthesia had been unwarranted.[18]

Tyler-Smith and Ramsbotham may have praised Simpson, but they used Snow's techniques. Ramsbotham maintained that Simpson's method "must be attended with no small amount of danger." Like many others, Ramsbotham found it safer and just as satisfactory to bring "the system partially under the influence," as Snow had suggested.[19]

The demonstration of the order and predictability of

anesthesia may have been Snow's most important contribution. He also developed better ways to administer anesthesia and showed others how they could use it safely. As others copied his methods, the rancor and rhetoric that had characterized early discussions of anesthesia subsided. Textbooks and clinical papers began to contain more observation and less dogma. Unfortunately, Snow had less impact on clinical thought than on clinical practice. Although physicians followed his recommendations, they did not appear to understand or appreciate the careful preparation behind Snow's work. Nor did they appreciate the extent to which Snow had used science to shape clinical practice. Their oversight may reflect the residual influence of French physicians and their distrust of theory and speculation. In any case, Snow's contemporaries failed to recognize the value of scientific methodology and depended on the accumulation of experience. Still facing them were several unresolved issues regarding anesthesia—its effects on the child, on the uterus, and on infection and its relation to maternal and fetal death.

The perspective that John Snow acquired during the course of a short career did not pass to the rest of the medical profession for almost half a century. Good work emerged, but it came from an entirely new direction. By 1880 the focus of medical innovation had shifted from hospitals in France to universities in Germany. German scientists excelled in physiology and chemistry, and German physicians learned how to incorporate scientific principles into clinical practice. They improved medical education, attracting the students who had previously flocked to Edinburgh and Paris. It was German clinicians who first demonstrated the potential effect of drugs on the unborn child.

CHAPTER FIVE

"The Tender Organization of the Newborn"

Balancing the Risks of Pain and Anesthesia

Even supposing that the progress of labour should have taken

place normally, both for mother and child, how can we, as yet,

know or ascertain the possible consequences of the use of such

an agent on the brain of the child? — and how can we calculate

what may be the ultimate consequences of its action in

reference to the development of the mental faculties?

— H. V. Malen, in the *Lancet,* 1848

Of the safety issues identified by Simpson, dealing with the effects of anesthesia on the newborn proved the most difficult to resolve. Concern for the newborn was something new. Until the nineteenth century the mortality rate of women in labor had been so high that survival of the mother had overshadowed almost all other problems, becoming the most important criterion for the success of clinical management. Obstetricians had little experience evaluating the newborn, much less relating its condition to pregnancy or labor. In 1862, when the first paper appeared in England that associated birthing problems with permanent damage, its subject was hailed as "an original field of observation."[1] Physicians, who were just learning to recognize the catastrophic sequelae of premature birth, asphyxia, and abnormal labor, may have found the effects of anesthesia on neonates a subtle, if not trivial, problem.

Compounding the practical problem of recognizing the effects of anesthesia on the infant was a theoretical difficulty. In 1847, the year of the first obstetric anesthetic, no one was certain that ether and chloroform actually crossed the placenta. Physiologists knew a lot about placental function but argued about the transfer of the respiratory gases. Many of them thought that oxygen and carbon dioxide did not cross and that physicians therefore had little reason to fear the intrauterine effects of chloroform or ether. Although the literature contained sufficient information to resolve the question, few physicians other than John Snow had considered the data or developed a way of tackling the problem. Observations that Snow made during the course of clinical work led him to several assumptions—all of them correct—about the placental transmission of gases. Having smelled ether on the breath of the newborn, he assumed that ether moved rapidly from mother to child. He deduced, correctly, that chloroform would behave the same way. Having observed that most newborns were alert, even when their mothers were drowsy from anesthesia, he suggested that the infant had received a smaller dose than its mother and that the placenta had imposed some delay. Noting, however, that deeply anesthetized women delivered sleepy, less reactive infants, he deduced that levels of anesthesia in the infant could increase were the mother to receive a larger dose for a longer period of time.[2]

Some physicians agreed with Snow. Francis Ramsbotham worried that ether might be "detrimental to the tender organization of the newborn," because he had twice observed that fetal heart rate increased on administration of ether and decreased on its discontinuation.[3] To him, this sequence suggested a direct effect of ether on the fetal heart. Ramsbotham and Snow based their opinions about placental transport not on speculation but on observation of clinical phenomena. As common as these effects are today, one wonders why so many early obstetricians failed to see them or to recognize their significance.

Clinical Evidence for Placental Transport Before 1850

Among those who failed to observe the phenomena and to comprehend their significance were Channing and Simpson. Channing discounted placental transfer because he could not smell ether at the ends of the freshly cut umbilical cord.[4] If he had smelled the breath of the newborn, as Snow did, he, too, would have detected ether. Its odor is strong on the exhalations of any recently anesthetized patient, something readily apparent to any physician who has ever administered the drug. Nor did Simpson take note of effects of anesthesia on the newborn. Disposed as he was to using a deep level of anesthesia for a long period of time, many of the children whom he delivered must have been sluggish or depressed. How did Channing and Simpson miss phenomena that were so apparent to others, and how did such a sharp division arise between those who recognized the potential dangers of anesthesia and those who did not?

Simpson's lapse is particularly strange because medical literature for centuries had taught that all variety of materials cross the placenta. Even the Greek philosopher Aristotle had said in his book on embryology that the placenta took nutrients from the mother's blood just as the roots of a tree took sustenance from the soil. In a book on embryology the Jacobean physician William Harvey, best known for correctly describing the dynamics of the circulatory system, repeated Aristotle's analogy. Coincidentally, John Mayow, an early Oxford physiologist, compared the placenta to a lung in that the placenta facilitated transfer of "nitro-aerial" particles from the mother's blood to the fetus. Two hundred years later, the physiologist W. B. Carpenter developed this idea, comparing the movement of nutrients from maternal to fetal blood to the movement of nutrients across the gastrointestinal mucosa into the veins and lacteals, a process that had been studied and documented rather well by 1850.[5]

Long before the discovery of bacteria, physicians had known of women who contracted smallpox or syphilis during pregnancy and then delivered infants who had the active disease. Other physicians had given phosphorus, mercury, lead, potassium iodide, or saffron to pregnant women only to find traces of these compounds in the organs or body fluids of the offspring. Noting bile-stained internal organs in infants born to women who later died of acute liver failure, physicians reasoned, correctly, that bile had moved from the mother's bloodstream to the infant's through the placenta. By 1850 clinical evidence for placental transport was sufficient to prompt the Scottish physician Alexander Harvey to write "On the Foetus in Utero, as Inoculating the Maternal with the Peculiarities of the Paternal Organism; and on Mental States in Either Parent, as Influencing Nutrition and Development of the Offspring," in which he gave convincing evidence to support his thesis. The paper, published in the *Edinburgh Journal of Medical Sciences,* was cited often in the United States and Great Britain and on the Continent and most certainly was known to Simpson.[6]

The data, both scientific and medical, shared a common problem, however. The evidence was not definitive. Reasonable though the assumption was that the placenta served the fetus as an organ of nutrition, or that it transferred nitro-aerial particles (oxygen, bile, smallpox, or whatever), reasonableness did not constitute proof. In a medical era dominated by French skepticism, physicians discounted the value of theory unsubstantiated by fact. Besides, they recognized that placental transmission of anesthetic gases was only one part of a complex problem: to show not only that drugs crossed the placenta but that they crossed quickly, that they caused damage, and that the detrimental effects of ether and chloroform on the fetus exceeded their benefits to the mother. Perhaps the unexpected complexity of the issue explains why it stymied clinicians for so long.

Two developments induced physicians to reconsider the problem of placental transfer. The first was a change in the use of opioids. The second was an intense interest in fetal and maternal metabolism that began in German universities and medical schools.

Although physicians had long administered opioids, they seldom prescribed them for childbirth. For one thing, there were technical problems. Until 1809 only crude extracts of opium had been available. Although these extracts were effective, the response of patients was often erratic and slow, partly because the preparations varied in purity but also because physicians had no reliable way to administer opioids. Patients in labor often vomit, so any opioid administered by mouth would be lost before it could be adsorbed through the wall of the stomach.

Two important technical innovations removed some of the uncertainty of giving opioids. In 1809 the German pharmacist Wilhelm Sertürner isolated morphine and codeine, two of opium's most active components. Using purified derivatives instead of crude extracts improved the predictability of the response. Equally important, physicians soon had a better way to administer the drug. By 1853 Alexander Wood had invented the hollow metal needle, and E. Pravaz had invented the syringe. Subcutaneous injection gave physicians a way to avoid the vagaries of gastrointestinal adsorption.[7]

Given the propensity of Victorians to innovate, physicians soon used morphine administered hypodermically for a bewildering variety of ailments—from renal stones and rheumatism to sexual dysfunction and psychoses. Inevitably, they also used it for obstetrics. In 1868 the German physician Ernst Kormann recommended hypodermic morphine for labor pain. Shortly thereafter, Isaac Taylor, a professor of obstetrics at the College of Physicians and Surgeons in New York City, introduced Kormann's method to American physicians. Effective, inexpensive, and easy to use, hypodermic injection of morphine had many advantages.[8]

Unfortunately, hypodermic morphine also had disadvantages. Obstetricians soon voiced many of the same objections to morphine that they had raised to ether and chloroform: that morphine would slow or stop labor, not an unreasonable assumption in the context of medical theory of that time, and that it would damage the child. As early as 1834, Francis Ramsbotham had warned that children born to addicted women were "dull and sleepy in the first hours of life." J. Pereira, in the 1842 edition of his popular pharmacology textbook, advised against giving opioids to pregnant or nursing women, saying that both the placenta and breast milk transmit the drugs to the child, which, he said, would impose significant risks, although he failed to say what those risks might be.[9]

Reinforcing medical concerns about opioids were growing problems related to the social use of such drugs. During the first half of the nineteenth century, few people recognized the addictive properties of opioids. With no laws limiting their use, opioids became a frequent component of patent medicines. Mothers even soothed their teething infants by rubbing morphine on their gums. The inevitable increase in rates of addiction had both social and medical consequences.[10]

As addiction increased in the general population, physicians identified more problems among obstetric patients. One French physician, concerned about a patient's large daily requirement for morphine, convinced her to take less. When she did, however, movements of the fetus became so violent that the physician feared she would abort. After she resumed her original dose, the fetus again became quiet. He assumed that the child had become addicted *in utero* and that he had observed fetal signs of withdrawal. Other physicians reported signs of opioid withdrawal in newborns or unexpected fetal death shortly after birth, purportedly because of hypodermic administration of morphine to the mother during labor. In medical meetings, physicians discussed these problems with a new urgency. Coincidentally, they began to reexamine experimental evidence dealing with placental transport.[11]

Experimental Evidence for Placental Transport

By 1850 evidence was mounting in favor of placental transmission of drugs. By injecting camphor into the circulation of pregnant dogs the French physiologist François Magendie had shown that the drug could travel to fetal organs. A description of this experiment appeared in an 1834 English translation of Magendie's textbook, copies of which were undoubtedly available to Channing and Simpson through medical libraries at their institutions. Similarly, the German physician W. Reitz had injected particles of mercuric sulfite into the circulation of pregnant rabbits. At the autopsy, he observed particles of the compound wedged in the small vessels of fetal brains. Two other physicians, F. A. Hoffmann and Paul Langerhans, repeated the experiment and were unable to duplicate Reitz's results, but an Englishman, W. S. Savory, found that strychnine injected into the circulation of fetal dogs caused the mother to convulse. From this, Savory concluded that the strychnine had crossed from the fetal blood through the placenta into the maternal bloodstream.[12]

The first person to test specifically for placental transfer of an anesthetic was C. C. Hüter, a professor of obstetrics at the University of Marburg. Having once smelled chloroform emanating from the liver of a stillborn child during an autopsy, Hüter worried that anesthetic gases might cross the placenta, have deleterious effects on the vascular and nervous systems of the infant, and predispose the child to depression or death. In 1850 he described his use of a chemical test to identify chloroform in the umbilical-cord blood of newborns. Hüter's studies should have alerted physicians

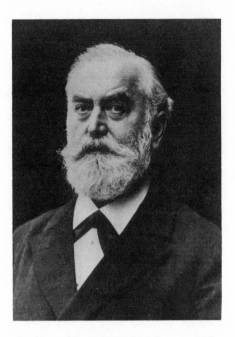

Paul Zweifel (1848–1927). Courtesy of
the Archiv für Gynaekologie, Berlin.

but did not. In fact, almost twenty-five years elapsed before
incontestable data settled the debate. The proof came from
work of a Swiss physician named Paul Zweifel.[13]

Zweifel, like Hüter, began with a clinical observation.
During studies of fetal metabolism, he had observed an unexpected chemical reaction in the urine of infants delivered
from women who had been given chloroform during labor.
The reaction resembled that produced by glucose, which
caused Zweifel to speculate that exposure to chloroform
during labor had altered the way the infant metabolized car-
bohydrates. It was Zweifel's interest in glucose that led him
to the problem of anesthesia.

In subsequent tests Zweifel learned that the substance

in question was not glucose, as he had originally assumed, but chloroform. Recognizing the clinical significance of his unexpected discovery, Zweifel published his research in 1874. Several people criticized his report because he had performed his tests on placental tissue. They said that the positive results could represent contamination by maternal blood adherent to the placental membranes. Zweifel laid such doubts to rest with publication of a second, more extensive paper.[14] Testing fetal blood and urine instead of the placenta, he again obtained a positive reaction for the presence of chloroform. He thus confirmed that chloroform does cross the placenta quickly, even during labor. To substantiate the rapidity of drug transfer, he showed that he could also detect salicylic acid in the urine of newborns after he administered it to the mother during labor (thereby replicating an experiment first performed by Benecke). Within a short time, others repeated and confirmed Zweifel's work. Definitive and reproducible, Zweifel's experiments ended debate: from 1877 on, no one seriously questioned the idea that anesthetic agents or any other drug might quickly cross the placenta.

German Preeminence in Medicine, 1850–1900

Zweifel's experiments, though well done, added little to what Hüter had shown twenty-five years earlier. But Zweifel's work had more impact because an important change had occurred in medicine. During the short interval between the two sets of experiments, the medical revolution that began in France during the first half of the century moved to Germany. Universities in Berlin, Leipzig, Tübingen, and Strassburg replaced the hospitals of Paris, Nancy, and Lyon as centers of medical education and innovation. One measure of the change was the number of foreigners who studied in

German medical schools during the last decades of the nineteenth century: by some estimates more than fifteen thousand Americans studied medicine in German schools between 1870 and 1914.[15]

The empiricism of the French physicians had run its course. Their distrust of theory and speculation had helped to dismantle Galenic medicine early in the century, but skepticism alone offered no basis for further growth. Believing that the order underlying natural phenomena would reveal itself without recourse to theory, French clinicians and scientists indulged in the perpetual collection of data. Even when exhaustive and exact, observation without hypotheses could not lead to understanding, and descriptions of disease, no matter how precise, would not improve medical care. Science, French physicians learned, requires not only the accumulation of data but also the development of theories that give data meaning. Not even Magendie's work escaped this criticism.

German physicians, on the other hand, excelled at theory. Earlier in the nineteenth century their love of theory had hindered their work in biology and medical science. Later, they learned to fuse their penchant for philosophy to their proficiency with experiments. The combination proved very effective. By 1840 M. J. Schleiden and Theodor Schwann had developed the cell theory of biology—the idea that the fundamental unit of the body is the cell and that cells of different types combine to form distinct types of tissues, each having a unique function. Soon pathologists such as Rudolf Virchow learned to apply concepts of cell structure and function to the study of disease. Following this lead, German physicians and scientists began a systematic study of the tissue and cellular responses to disease and healing. At the same time, Johannes Müller and Karl Ludwig developed new concepts and methods of experimental physiology; Justus von Liebig and Felix Hoppe-Seyler laid the foundations of modern biochemistry; and Rudolf Buchheim and Oswald Schmiedeberg transformed herbal medicine into pharmacology. These scientists did not dismiss the Gallic distrust of speculation but instead showed how to test theory and keep it within bounds through experimentation. The approach that they developed became the basis for a new style of medical practice, one that is still useful. Principles of chemistry and anatomy, of cellular, tissue, and organ physiology, replaced the humors of Galen as the basis for medical practice.

Contributing to the success of German physicians was the status given them by the public. Unlike in England, France, and the United States, where physicians trained in independent hospitals, proprietary schools, or apprenticeships, in Germany medical schools were established at universities. Even more important, German universities required their medical faculty and students to meet the same high standards of scholarship as members of other university departments. Simply practicing medicine and lecturing did not suffice. To secure promotion the faculty also had to perform scholarly work, and the universities gave generous support toward this end. At a time when two of France's best-known physician-scientists, Louis Pasteur and Claude Bernard, barely had the resources to carry out their work, German laboratories were well equipped and staffed.

Foreign students in Germany observed the conditions contributing to the success of German schools. Whenever possible they took German methods of teaching and research to their medical institutions at home. As a consequence, there developed an international cadre of physicians who were sophisticated and well trained in science. The number of such physicians remained small, however, and most practiced in a handful of prestigious schools, such as Johns Hopkins. However, medicine was changing. Zweifel addressed a more knowledgeable group of physicians than Hüter had just a quarter of a century before.

The Experiments of Gusserow and Zweifel

Swiss born, Paul Zweifel (1848–1927), the third generation in his family to become a physician, studied medicine in Zurich. After graduation, he studied with Adolf Gusserow (1836–1906), a German and one of Europe's foremost obstetricians. After the Franco-Prussian War of 1870–1871, Gusserow and many other German academics were appointed to posts at the University of Strassburg in Alsace-Lorraine. Zweifel followed his professor to Strassburg, where he conducted his experiments with chloroform, extending a line of research started by Gusserow using methods developed by Felix Hoppe-Seyler, another prominent member of the Strassburg faculty.[16] Undoubtedly, Zweifel's close association with Gusserow, Hoppe-Seyler, and other members of that distinguished faculty contributed greatly to his success.

Gusserow, Zweifel's mentor, had a strong interest in fetal metabolism, particularly in the placental transfer of nutrients required for normal growth and development. For physiologists this was an old problem, but Gusserow recognized that it also had important clinical implications. Years earlier, the renowned physiologist Johannes Müller had suggested that the fetus itself consumed little or no oxygen in its own tissues, relying instead on the metabolic processes of the mother. Müller had reached this conclusion because he had failed to detect a difference in the oxygen content of arterial and venous blood in the umbilical cord. Gusserow knew of

Müller's experiments and had discussed them in several of his own papers.[17]

Gusserow wished to test Müller's theory, in particular the idea that fetal tissue cannot metabolize materials for itself. Resolution of the issue depended in part on estimates of the rate of transfer of various compounds across the placenta. A paper published in 1871 described experiments in which Gusserow had estimated the speed of transfer of potassium iodide and salicylic acid, compounds normally given to women during the last weeks of pregnancy or during labor. After his patients delivered, Gusserow analyzed samples of amniotic fluid and the urine of the newborns. The very small amounts of the drugs that he was able to recover suggested to him that placental transfer was too slow a process to support independent fetal metabolism. Thus, his initial data lent support to Müller's theory.[18]

When Gusserow reexamined the problem in 1878, he used an ingenious new test to detect fetal metabolism. Knowing that the kidney transforms benzoic acid into hippuric acid during passage of the drug from the circulation into the urine, Gusserow administered benzoic acid to pregnant women. (Presumably, he learned of this reaction from Oswald Schmiedeberg, the person who originally described it. Schmiedeberg, who was also on the faculty at Strassburg, was one of the founders of modern pharmacology.) When Gusserow found hippuric acid in the urine of the newborn children, he inferred that the benzoic acid had traversed the placenta and that the fetal kidney itself had transformed (metabolized) the drug independently of any action by the mother. These data contradicted his earlier experiments and called Müller's theory into question.[19]

Zweifel's experiments of 1874–1876 were an extension

of Gusserow's work and a further test of Müller's theory. Zweifel established that oxygen crosses the placenta by comparing the amount of oxygen contained in arterial and venous blood from the umbilical cord.[20] For this experiment he used a biophysical method perfected and popularized by Felix Hoppe-Seyler, the professor of physiologic chemistry at Strassburg. Hoppe-Seyler, already famous for his research and for founding one of the world's first journals of biochemistry, had shown that the spectral bands of light reflected from the surface of blood shift when oxygen combines with hemoglobin. Simply put, blood turns from dark to bright red as it absorbs oxygen. Using this spectral light absorption technique, Zweifel demonstrated that blood flowing from the fetus to the placenta contains less oxygen than blood flowing from the placenta back to the fetus. That such an experiment should have been necessary is curious, because the difference in color can easily be seen with the naked eye, a fact already known to any obstetrician who had looked carefully at the umbilical cord. Nevertheless, Zweifel's experiment convinced skeptics. His work proved that the fetus consumed oxygen and that the placenta transferred oxygen at a rate sufficient to supply the metabolic requirements of the fetus. Zweifel's studies of chloroform published in 1877 confirmed what he had already shown for oxygen. His papers were widely circulated. Physiologists as well as clinicians discussed them.[21]

Between 1850 and 1875 medicine changed. In 1850 Channing and Simpson had argued about the placental transfer of anesthetics, and Snow had accepted the fact of transfer based on clinical observation. Just twenty-five years later, Zweifel proved placental transfer by means of sophisticated chemical and physical tests.

Zweifel had more than ingenuity and perseverance. He had the good fortune to study and work with Adolf Gusserow, a clinician with a strong interest in fetal metabolism and a vision of its relevance to clinical practice. Zweifel also had the luck to be in Strassburg when the faculty of the medical school had many eminent clinical scientists of the caliber of Hoppe-Seyler and Schmiedeberg.

Conditions in Strassburg were not unique. Throughout Germany other scientists and clinicians worked on related problems, such as the energetics of growth and development, physiologic chemistry, and nutrition. By the end of the century physicians and scientists had also learned much about placental transport and fetal metabolism. They had created detailed descriptions of the microscopic anatomy of the uterus and placenta, including comparative studies of different species. They had estimates of rates of blood flow through uterine and umbilical circulatory systems, measurements of the oxygen and carbon dioxide used by the fetus, as well as studies of the relation between the chemical characteristics of compounds and their movement across the placenta. All of this was highly technical and intellectually sophisticated work, and it was all considered an integral part of clinical medicine.

Despite the quality of and widespread interest in Zweifel's work, his experiments had relatively little impact on practice, in part because many obstetricians had modified their use of anesthesia even before publication of Zweifel's papers. When they abandoned Simpson's method for Snow's, they limited fetal exposure to anesthetics and concomitantly diminished the risks. This made detecting the neonatal effects of anesthesia more difficult; it also made it less important. One physician said that he had thirty years of mostly quite satisfactory experience with anesthetics, and he saw no reason to modify his practice simply because Zweifel had shown that drugs cross the placenta.[22]

The response to Zweifel's work illustrates the gap that had developed between practicing physicians and clinical scientists. It was one thing to make an important new discovery. It was another to understand the implications of the discovery and learn how to apply it to clinical practice. Zwiefel's experiments also illustrate the disparity between obstetric practice in Germany and elsewhere. Obstetric journals published in England and America lacked the sophistication and polish of their German counterparts. Teaching in those two countries also lagged: as late as 1900 some medical schools still did not require training in obstetrics for graduation. Even though general practitioners delivered more babies than specialists, many students in both countries graduated from medical school without ever having attended a delivery. Throughout the nineteenth century and even into the twentieth, physicians in Great Britain and the United States, eager to raise the prestige of their profession, worked hard to distinguish obstetrics from midwifery.

The increasing technical and scientific complexity of obstetric practice that began in Germany during the last half of the nineteenth century began to increase the distance between physicians and patients. However crude and inaccurate, most patients could understand the principles of Galenic medicine. When physiology, pharmacology, chemistry, pathology, and bacteriology became the basis for practice, few members of the lay public had either the training or the experience to understand the pathogenesis, diagnosis, or treatment of disease. As this gap widened, physicians found themselves trying to find common ground between two different perceptions of pain and disease, that of the scientists and that of the public. Accordingly, patients and physicians often disagreed, particularly with respect to the management of childbirth pain. Conflicts between medical science and social values became a recurrent theme during most of the twentieth century.

PART II

Women and the Pain of Childbirth

"The Sin of Our First Parents"

The Social Connotations of Pain

Lett us, Look upon Sin as the Cause of Sickness.

There are it may be, Two Thousand Sicknesses:

And indeed, any one of whom able to crush us!

But what is the Cause of all? Bear in Mind,

That Sin was that which first brought sickness

upon a Sinful World, and which yett continues

to Sicken the World, with a World of Diseases.

Sickness is in short, Flagellum Dei pro pecatis Mundi;

First, Remember, That the Sin of our First Parents,

was the First Parent of all our Sickness.

—Cotton Mather, *The Angel of Bethesda,* circa 1724

Underlying the controversy about anesthesia for childbirth was the problem of pain itself. Ether anesthesia gave physicians the power to obliterate pain. It also forced them to learn more about pain's biology: What constitutes a painful stimulus? How does the nervous system perceive pain? How does pain affect the rest of the body? Does pain have a biological function? Is pain part of disease, or is it part of healing? Is pain inevitable? Is there life without pain? If an individual ceases to feel pain, does that person die? Although some of these questions bordered on philosophy, physicians needed answers if they were to balance the risks of pain against the risks of anesthesia. Establishing the balance, which the historian Martin Pernick labeled a "calculus of suffering," proved a formidable task.[1]

Pernick suggests that the calculus of suffering formulated by physicians included cultural as well as medical considerations. Treating pain was not simply an exercise in choosing the best drug or the most appropriate dose. It also meant deciding which patients should be treated and identifying the circumstances in which treatment was appropriate. Often these decisions impinged on social issues: Who feels pain? Do some individuals or groups feel pain more intensely than others? Are all people equally deserving of pain relief? Do pain and suffering have social consequences independent of their effects on the body? Does pain influence the development of the individual or the formation of social bonds? Such questions, which went far beyond medical practice, could not be resolved by ever more detailed studies of physiology, anatomy, or pharmacology. In fact, physicians were no better qualified to answer these questions than were their patients.

The social issues that influenced the development of

the calculus had another important characteristic. Unlike the medical questions, which surfaced only after physicians applied anesthesia, the cultural factors had a history that extended back to antiquity. Medical practice had grown out of that cultural tradition and been shaped by it. Anesthesia could develop and survive only in a culture that valued the relief of pain.

Culture and the Response to Pain

The public rejected the idea of anesthesia several times in the nineteenth century before it caught on. Drugs capable of inducing anesthesia were available almost fifty years before Morton's successful demonstration of ether anesthesia in Boston. Prominent scientists had even suggested that such drugs be used for that purpose. By 1824 Sir Humphry Davy had recognized the anesthetic properties of nitrous oxide. His student Michael Faraday had commented on the soporific effects of ether, and Henry Hill Hickman had suggested that carbon dioxide be used as an anesthetic. By 1844 an American physician, Crawford Long, had successfully used ether to anesthetize a patient for surgery, although he failed to publicize his accomplishment, and Horace Wells had tried to do the same with nitrous oxide, although his public demonstration failed. Countless others had used ether and nitrous oxide for "frolics." Yet no one had established the idea that drugs could, and should, be given to patients to free them of surgical pain. In fact, each of these men encountered some form of opposition: Davy from an uninterested patron, Faraday and Hickman from the scientific community, and Wells from skeptical surgeons. Crawford Long's situation is particularly interesting. Inhabitants of his hometown,

Jefferson, Georgia, almost ostracized him. Patients under-
going surgery felt less threatened by hypnosis than by ether.[2]
Opposition had disappeared by 1846, the year the public embraced the idea of anesthesia. The effusive response
to Morton's experiment stimulated Jacob Bigelow, a surgeon
who had observed the demonstration in the ether dome, to
remark, "No single announcement ever created so great and
general excitement in so short a time. Surgeons, sufferers,
scientific men, everybody, united in simultaneous demonstrations of heartfelt mutual congratulation."

Within another fifty years physicians would discover the
analgesic properties of aspirin and the ability of cocaine to
induce local anesthesia. Reflecting on public response to
these and other medical discoveries, William James wrote: "A
strange moral transformation has, within the past century,
swept over our Western world. We no longer think that we
are called on to face physical pain with equanimity. . . . The
way in which our ancestors looked upon pain as an eternal
ingredient of the world's order, and both caused and suffered it as a matter-of-course portion of their day's work, fills
us with amazement."[3]

James was more struck by the transformation in the social perception of pain than by the discovery of a medical
method to treat pain. Nor was he alone in his response. Historian Owen Chadwick once described the early nineteenth
century as an era when Western society willingly jettisoned
many ideas that it had once believed essential to its very existence.[4] In other words, ether, aspirin, and cocaine were less
a cause of the revolution in the public perception of pain
and suffering than a product of it. For the most part, the
social transformation was complete before the discovery of
any of these pharmacologic agents.

The traditions of pain that the public jettisoned in the nineteenth century arose from among the ancient Greeks and Jews. Attitudes toward pain influenced many aspects of life in both groups. The historian J. J. Pollitt suggests that the art and philosophy of the ancient Greeks represented their attempt to cope with the chaotic suffering and brutality of their lives. In an even more expansive comment, the Catholic theologian E. Schillebeeckx suggests that "the history of suffering among men, and indeed in the animal world and throughout the universe, is a constant theme of every account of life, every philosophy and every religion." Another writer, C. S. Lewis, succinctly notes "that all great religions were first preached and long practiced, in a world without chloroform."[5] These comments do not imply that art, philosophy, and religion relieved physical pain but rather that efforts to mitigate pain and suffering are pervasive and may take many forms.

Notable in both the Jewish and the Greek traditions was the frequent association of pain with sin and divine punishment. Best known, perhaps, is the Old Testament story of Adam and Eve, but other examples abound.[6] In the Book of Job we read: "The wicked man travaileth with pain all his days" (5:17); "he is chastened also with pain upon his bed and the multitude of his bones with strong pain so that his life abhorreth bread and his soul dainty meat" (33:19–20). Comparable passages appear in Isaiah (3:10–11), Genesis (38:7), and Psalms (92:6–8). Groups of sinners, like the inhabitants of Sodom and Gomorrah, are punished by pestilence or total destruction. In contrast, righteousness may confer immunity (Proverbs 12:21). In one respect, the story of Job seems inconsistent with this theology, because Job was a righteous man, but the story makes the point because the "comforters" interpreted Job's misfortune as de facto evidence of prior sin.

Greek epics and plays also emphasized the divine origin of pain and suffering. In *The Odyssey*, Zeus says, "My word, how mortals take the gods to task! All their afflictions come from us, we hear." In *The Oresteia*, Aeschylus writes, "Every mortal who outraged god or guest or loving parent; each receives the pain his pains exact." It is for this reason that the gods punished Prometheus for stealing fire and Pandora for opening the box.[7]

Early Christian concepts of the origin of pain and disease resembled many of their Greek and Jewish antecedents. The Gospel of John (5:14) describes how Christ admonished a man whom he had just healed: "Behold, thou art made whole: sin no more, lest a worse thing come unto thee." Early theologians did have some difficulty reconciling the existence of suffering with their concept of a good and loving God. From the fifth century on, they often deferred to St. Augustine, who affirmed the inherent evil of humankind and the enslavement to sin as a legacy from Adam and Eve.[8]

Naturally enough, many religious conventions regarding pain spilled over into secular life. Boccaccio, author of *The Decameron*, ascribed the bubonic plague to "God's just anger with our wicked deeds sent . . . as a punishment to mortal men . . . [which] no doctor's advice, no medicine could overcome or alleviate." Secular organizations used pain to establish order in the community in the same way and for the same reason as the gods in traditional stories. The infliction of pain was an integral part of the legal system. Torture was sanctioned to extract information and confessions, and brutal executions were staged to punish but also to edify and entertain the public. The English words *pain* and *patient* preserve this tradition, derived as they are from the Latin *poena* and *patior,* which mean "punish" and "endure." Some have suggested that public spectacles of pain inured people to suffering and contributed to the atmosphere of resignation that prevailed in the Middle Ages.[9]

Embedded in Greek, Jewish, and Christian traditions was the idea that pain might even offer benefits. The pain that punished could also purify. Christianity, in particular, emphasized the redemptive value of pain. The ultimate Christian symbol of pain, the cross, became a metaphor for sacrifice, forgiveness, and salvation: "For since by man came death, by man came also the resurrection of the dead. For as in Adam all die, even so in Christ shall all be made alive" (1 Corinthians 15:21-22). On this basis, the cross became a pervasive theme in art and literature, a symbol that the Crusaders carried to the Middle East, and conquistadors, to the Americas. The cross even acquired special powers—among them the ability to conquer evil spirits and to cure.[10]

Religious connotations of pain influenced social behavior. Ascetics used self-flagellation and self-mutilation as acts of atonement. During epidemics of bubonic plague, flagellants hoped that their plight would move God to spare them worse pain or even death.

Pain could also bestow special status. One historian, Peter Brown, notes religious ascetics in early Christian communities used pain and suffering to create for themselves a unique social position as the physical representative of the seen and the unseen worlds—the junction, as it were, of earth and heaven. According to Brown, the lifestyle of these Holy Men, characterized by "prolonged and clearly visible rituals of self mortification," earned them respect and secular power. They became "dead" to the world, a state that enabled them to take action when others could not, as mediators in disputes among communities, for example. During the Middle Ages, Christians and Muslims alike believed that wounds sustained in righteous battle would guarantee them preferential treatment in the afterlife. In the tenth-century lyric poem *The Song of Roland*, the archbishop says to his soldiers, who are outnumbered by infidels and clearly close to death, "It is far better for us to die fighting. . . . Holy paradise is open to you. You will take your seat amongst the Innocents." Depictions of such events through stories, poems, plays, and art have helped perpetuate the belief that suffering incurred for the public good has social value.[11]

Religious explanations of pain had practical results. Apart from supplying a rationale for pain, religion offered physical relief by encouraging the formation of organizations for dispensing care. This, too, reflected early theology. Jewish and Christian tradition taught that the God who punished also healed: "He maketh sore and bindeth up: he woundeth, and his hands make whole" (Job 5:17–18). God, the ultimate source of all healing, conferred on rabbis, his earthly representatives, the power to purify. This tradition invested priests and, later, physicians with great status, authority, and responsibility. Apart from overseeing the spiritual and physical needs of those who came to them, they also became responsible for public health measures, as outlined in the Book of Leviticus. Insofar as disease was a manifestation of a sick soul, spiritual healing became a prerequisite for a bodily cure. Christ had transferred his healing powers to the apostles, and they delegated this power to the church. Early Christians, therefore, practiced medicine as an act of faith, as well as an act of mercy.[12]

During the Middle Ages, as the Christian church grew in wealth and power, its medical work became better organized. Such groups as the Orders of Lazarus and of Benedictus assumed care of the sick as part of their ministry. Two better-known orders, the Knights Templar and the Knights of the Hospital of St. John, started out with the same mission but became more militant. Theologians devised special prayers and liturgies for the sick and dying, and caring for sick parishioners became an important religious activity for the clergy.

With the expansion of medical care by the church, the practice of medicine acquired religious overtones. Individuals were canonized for their work among the sick—Damian, Cosmos, Elizabeth of Hungary—and architects incorporated religious metaphors, such as the cross, into the design of Europe's first hospitals. The involvement of the church also reinforced the idea that every member of the community was responsible for the less fortunate.

As naturalistic philosophies replaced religion during the Renaissance and Enlightenment there was some modification of the traditional explanations of pain and disease. Ministers of religion continued to perform medical functions, but now they used a different rationale. Instead of arguing that disease, pain, and suffering were personally inflicted by God, they presented pain and suffering as phenomena that obeyed natural laws. Instead of asserting that their mission to heal was a direct charge from God, they claimed that their superior education made them the group best prepared to interpret natural law—a rationale that helped keep the functions of priest and physician combined, particularly in northern Europe. Immigrants carried this tradition to the Americas. The first president of the Medical Society of New Jersey (1766) was a minister as well as a physician, as were six of the other thirty-six founding members of the group. In fact, some early ministers are best known for their scientific and medical work. Joseph Priestley studied oxygen, and Stephen Hales was the first to measure blood pressure. In succeeding decades, the study of the biology of the disease would replace theology altogether. During the era immediately before the introduction of anesthesia, however, theology and medicine remained intertwined.[13]

The union of religion and medicine continued in colonial America, as exemplified by two books, one by Cotton Mather and the other by John Wesley (1703–1791). Mather (1663–1728), a prominent Puritan minister who served as one of the judges at the Salem witch trials, also knew medicine. He helped to introduce inoculation as a method to control smallpox and even encouraged a statistical study to evaluate its worth. Mather was curious, well educated, and extremely well read. His personal library contained more than six hundred books, an exceptional number for that time and place. After consulting 250-plus references, Mather wrote a medical textbook, *The Angel of Bethesda.* Though not published during his lifetime, it reflects both the theology and the medicine of the day. *Primitive Remedies,* written by John Wesley, founder of Methodism, became popular throughout the American colonies before the Revolutionary War.[14]

Each book listed folk remedies for such common problems as stomachache, bee sting, toothache, and kidney stones. Interspersed with medical advice was a generous serving of traditional Christian theology. Commenting on the origin of disease, for example, Wesley wrote, "As he knew no sin, so he knew no pain, no sickness, weakness or bodily disorder. . . . The entire creation was at peace with man, so long as man was at peace with his Creator." Cotton Mather laced his medicine with even larger doses of theology. "Now,

Sickness is to awaken our Concern, first, for the Pardon of the Maladies in our souls. . . . Lord, look upon my Affliction and my Pain, and forgive all my Sin." [15]

The traditions of pain and suffering that permeated philosophy, law, social custom, and religion appeared, of course, in the social response to childbirth. Eve's fall from grace in the Garden of Eden was considered the beginning of problems for succeeding generations of women. The association of sex with sin and punishment in this story was perpetuated by theologians like St. Augustine. With very little modification the same ideas appeared in the writings of Cotton Mather twenty centuries later.

Mather exhorted women in labor to "Remember that Wormwood and Gall of the Forbidden Fruit; Lett your Soul have them still in Remembrance, and be humbled in you. Under all your Ails, think, The Sin of my Mother, which is also my Sin, has brought all this upon me! 'Harken to the councils of God'; consider the offspring a blessing; prepare for death and confess their sins." [16] He also suggested that women might find solace during labor by reflecting on a passage from 1 Timothy (2:15): "She shall be Saved in Childbearing if they continue in Faith, and Charity, and Holiness, with Sobriety." Only when theological reflection failed did Mather resort to such practical remedies as preparations of the "livers and galls of Eeles, dried slowly in an Oven," or "Date-Stones, Amber, Saffron, and Cummin-seeds" given "when the poor Woman is in her Extremity." Mercifully, for "Hard Labours of Women" he relented and recommended morphine.

Placing on patients the responsibility for difficult or painful labors was not just an idiosyncrasy of Christianity. Even the Greek physician Soranus of Ephesus (first century C.E.) had blamed idle habits, ignorance, denial, and excessive anxiety for many of the difficulties that women experienced during childbirth.[17]

Associated with the theology of childbirth was an air of resignation, if not despair. The poet John Donne (1572–1631), who studied medicine before he became a minister, wrote:

> There is no health: physicians say that we
> At best, enjoy but a neutrality.
> And can there be worse sickness, than to know
> That we are never well, nor can be so?
> We are born ruinous: poor mothers cry,
> That children come not right, nor orderly,
> Except they headlong come, and fall upon
> An ominous precipitation.[18]

Anne Bradstreet, a contemporary of Donne's and a Puritan compatriot of Mather's, echoed these feelings in "Before the Birth of One of Her Children," a poem that she addressed to her husband:

> All things within this fading world hath end,
> Adversity doth still our joyes attend;
> No tyes so strong, no friend so dear and sweet,
> But with death's parting blow is sure to meet.
> The sentence past is most irrevocable,
> A common thing, yet oh inevitable;
> How soon, My Dear, death may my steps attend,
> How soon't may be thy Lot to lose thy friend.

Bradstreet, like many of her contemporaries, witnessed such deaths in her own family. In another poem, she memorialized a daughter-in-law who died in childbirth and the grandchild who died at the same time. For pregnant women some measure of resignation was appropriate, if not necessary.

In addition to the certainty of pain during labor, they also faced the ever present prospect of death. Women with pelvic bones deformed by rickets or tuberculosis could expect a long painful labor, often followed by death. Overall, one in ten women died during childbirth. During epidemics in the nineteenth century puerperal fever sometimes killed as many as one in two. Pain and death were always close.[19]

The theological connotations of pain and disease prompted more direct church involvement in childbirth. The Anglican cleric Thomas Cranmer (1489–1556) included in his *Book of Common Prayer* a special service for women who had survived the rigors of childbirth. The service followed traditional doctrine, attributing pain to sin but praising God for his mercy in sparing the parturient death and the "pangs of hell." For a time in England and in France authority for licensure of midwives even lay with church officials, not with physicians. Their concern was not for the midwife's medical skills but for her qualifications to administer the last rites to the mother and baptize the child should either die before the arrival of a priest. Only after the Enlightenment did secular authorities assume responsibility for evaluating a midwife's medical training and technical proficiency.[20]

Before the introduction of modern anesthesia, strong and pervasive traditions invested pain, suffering, disease, and death with special meaning. The social and medical response to childbirth and its pain was part of this tradition. On the one hand, pain and suffering signified sin and punishment. For people taught to believe in the inherent evil of human beings, pain probably seemed unavoidable. But pain also signified sacrifice, a means to achieve redemption, a path to find God, and, on a more practical level, a mechanism to establish status or power within a secular community. Although pain could be a destructive experience, it could have social and spiritual value. From this tradition grew organizations that gave practical support to those in pain or need, such as hospitals and charitable societies.

Ironically, the success of the religious interpretations of pain, suffering, and disease may have slowed the development of secular medicine. Some historians have suggested that attributing to God the sole power to inflict pain and dispense healing relieved people of that responsibility. James Young Simpson appears to have been aware of this tradition, and it was frustration with public apathy in the face of pain and suffering that appears to have prompted him to write his well-known rebuttal.

Simpson and the Religious Interpretation of Pain

In December 1847, just eleven months after administering the first obstetric anesthetic, Simpson published a pamphlet entitled *Answers to the Religious Objections Advanced Against the Employment of Anaesthetic Agents in Midwifery and Surgery and Obstetrics.* Seven months later, he readdressed the subject in a long letter to Dr. Protheroe Smith, a London obstetrician who had written a similar pamphlet. Simpson described his dismay when he learned how "patients and others strongly object to the superinduction of anaesthesia in labour, by the inhalation of ether or chloroform, on the assumed ground that an immunity from pain during parturition was contrary to religion and the express command of the Scripture." The scriptural command in question was the passage from the Book of Genesis in which God condemned Eve's descendants to suffer during labor because of her disobedience in Eden. In the pamphlet Simpson launched a many-pronged attack against this teaching.[21]

Simpson began his argument by acknowledging the

Book of Genesis as the source of objections to using anesthesia for amelioration of pain. He also noted, however, that God himself had promised to remove the curse from Adam and Eve's descendants. Simpson said that traditional interpretations of the story were wrong. According to him, the phrase commonly translated "in sorrow thou shalt bring forth children" did not mean that women were to experience pain but that they were "to work" during childbirth. As used in the original text, Simpson said, the key word was ambiguous. Had the original author truly meant "pain," surely he would have chosen a different word, or so Simpson reasoned.

Simpson next sought to divest the pain of childbirth of its religious significance. The pain is an effect of anatomy, he argued, not an expression of divine wrath. An upright posture necessitated strong muscles in the floor of the pelvis to support the contents of the abdomen. To overcome this resistance during labor, the uterine muscle also had to be correspondingly stronger. The pressures generated by such a strong uterus caused pain and were a manifestation of a biological necessity.

Simpson proceeded to point out that God's curse had also included Adam, but this had never deterred men from adopting improvements in agriculture or transportation to ease the burden of physical labor. Therefore, he said, chastisement by God should not keep women from easing the pain of childbirth. In a final flourish, he pointed out that God himself had used anesthesia when he caused a "deep sleep" to fall over Adam so that he might extract the rib that would become Eve. Besides, Simpson said, God never would have given humans the intelligence to discover anesthesia had he not intended that they use it.

Simpson's foray into theology evoked some criticism. In

a letter published in the *Lancet,* physician Samuel Ashwell commented on the "impiety of making Jehovah an operating surgeon, and the absurdity of supposing that anaesthesia would be necessary in His hands." Ashwell also caught Simpson on a theological point, mentioning that "the deep sleep of Adam took place before the introduction of pain into the world during his state of innocence," which meant that Adam had had no need for anesthesia in Eden.[22]

Apart from niggling criticism, Simpson claimed that he had "received a variety of written and verbal communications from some of the best theologians and most esteemed clergymen here and elsewhere, and of all churches—Presbyterian, Independent, Episcopalian, etc.—approving of the views which I had taken." Even if we discount Simpson's proclivity for self-promotion, his observation seems accurate. Many physicians also commented favorably, including some who originally had opposed obstetric anesthesia on medical grounds.

Since 1847 many historians of medicine have claimed that Simpson's pamphlet marked a turning point in the public's acceptance of obstetric anesthesia and that it was as important as Queen Victoria's decision to have ether for her last two deliveries. Recently, however, A. D. Farr has challenged the importance of Simpson's pamphlet and his reinterpretation of the Adam and Eve story. Had Simpson's contemporaries still adhered to traditional religious interpretations of pain, they never would have accepted Simpson's arguments so readily. To test his idea, Farr searched medical journals, periodicals, newspapers, and official church documents. He found no evidence of opposition to obstetric anesthesia on religious grounds from either physicians or churchmen. He did learn that Simpson wrote his pamphlet in response to a rumor that a Liverpool surgeon, A. S. Parkes, intended to attack the medicinal use of anesthesia in a speech at a medical meeting. Farr points out, however, that minutes of the meeting contain no mention of the issue. Farr also suggests that stories of church opposition to anesthesia were more myth than fact. When questioned on the subject, Thomas Chalmers, a contemporary of Simpson's and a moderator of the Free Church of Scotland, said that he considered the origin of the pain of childbirth to be an issue for "small theologians."[23]

Farr suggests that stories of religious controversy originated with Simpson's daughter and with J. Duns, Simpson's biographer. He points out that Duns's biography contains no documentation, and that Simpson's daughter was very young when the pamphlet was published and probably had no personal knowledge of surrounding events other than family stories. In retrospect, it seems possible that Simpson sensed an opportunity and seized it. Certainly, this is in accord with his talent for creating news and eliciting public support. But even if true, this does not account for the historical persistence of the religious debate, which resurfaced in 1957, when the issue was thought to be of sufficient importance to be addressed by Pope Pius XII.

The importance of traditional interpretations of pain and suffering is beyond question. As Farr suggests, however, it seems improbable that Simpson's pamphlet would have been so popular had the majority of patients and physicians still adhered to the old views. More likely, Simpson gave voice to ideas that were already circulating among the public. But if so, we are left trying to explain the reluctance to use anesthesia that frustrated Simpson.

Most people—physicians and patients alike—probably did not blur the distinction between surgery and childbirth as Simpson did. To most people, surgery meant disease or a life-threatening injury. In such circumstances, the balance between risk and benefit—the calculus— must have seemed rather straightforward. In 1850, despite maternal mortality rates that were high by present-day standards, most physicians and large segments of the public still considered childbirth to be natural, not, as with cases for surgery, unnatural, making the risks of anesthesia seem high.

Public response to anesthesia has continued to vary with the perception of childbirth. When it is considered "natural," women criticize the administration of drugs. When they think childbirth "pathologic," they demand anesthesia. Developing a uniform and consistent calculus of suffering in the face of such variation has proved difficult.

Complicating the development of a calculus was the strange moral transformation that William James noted in 1901. Between the beginning and the end of the nineteenth century Western society began to look upon pain and suffering in new ways. This instigated a major change in the organization and function of many social institutions. Modern medicine was an outgrowth of this movement, and so was anesthesia. Eventually this movement even influenced the medical and social response to the pain of childbirth.

CHAPTER SEVEN

"This Blessed Chloroform"

Pain as Biological and Anesthesia as Necessary

The American Revolution, the forerunner of political changes

of the greatest character in Europe as well as in America, was

coincident with this new departure in medicine. . . . The faith of

Christendom has been, and is, crystallizing into new forms and

moving to new issues. It is not an extravagant assertion to say

that in all this turmoil, change and progress medicine has kept

abreast of the other natural sciences, of politics and of theology

and has made equal conquests over authority, error and

tradition. . . . Such has been the progress . . . and . . .

achievements of medical science. . . . To justify the enthusiastic

regard in which physicians hold their profession and to

deserve the gratitude of mankind.

—Edward H. Clarke, "Practical Medicine," 1876

With the revolution in economic, political, and religious thought that occurred in the first part of the nineteenth century, western Europeans and Americans developed a new understanding of themselves and of their relationship to the world around them. They rebelled against conditions they had once accepted passively, and changed situations they had once thought permanent. They valued the individual person more highly and looked for ways to improve daily life. Problems were approached with vigor and optimism, sometimes with little regard for the consequences of change.

Along with everything else, people rebelled against suffering and pain; science and technology would abolish these problems, they believed. Individuals would benefit from scientific progress, society would more nearly approach the utopian, and life would be better all around. These new beliefs affected the development of medicine and anesthesia, particularly with regard to childbirth, an area in which personal, cultural, and social considerations had always carried great weight.

Of the physicians involved in the debates, Simpson may have best understood the impact of the new social values on the practice of obstetrics—which may explain why in his campaign to establish obstetric anesthesia he bypassed the medical establishment and spoke directly to patients. Soon after he administered the first obstetric anesthetic he said, "Medical men may oppose for a time the superinduction of anaesthesia in parturition, but they will oppose it in vain; for certainly our patients themselves will force use of it upon the profession. The whole question is, even now, one, merely of time."[1] Cultural events of the preceding century had prepared patients to be receptive. By 1847 the public was so convinced that obstetric pain was unnecessary, if not dangerous, that the risks of anesthesia may have appeared trivial. Even though most physicians still feared anesthesia and spoke against it, public pressure forced its use. Social factors entered into the calculus of suffering.

Three cultural trends influenced the public: a change in the religious connotation of obstetric pain, the belief that the physical intensity of obstetric pain had increased, and a spirit of optimism and overwhelming faith that science and technology could overcome any problem. These factors still influence the practice of medicine.

The Declining Influence of the Church

As scientists and physicians relied more on observations and experiments for information and insight, intellectuals of the Enlightenment came to question the reliability of divine revelation and to challenge and discard many old ideas. Two traditional beliefs that fell from favor were the ideas that God had a punitive nature and man a sinful nature. Sometime during the Enlightenment, the stern, vengeful God of the Old Testament became the sympathetic and forgiving, albeit detached, God of the New Testament. A poem by William Blake (1757–1827) presents God's new image.

Think not, thou canst sigh a sigh,
And thy maker is not by.
Think not, thou canst weep a tear,
And thy maker is not near.
O! he gives to us his joy,
That our grief he may destroy

> Till our grief is fled and gone
> He doth sit by us and moan.

Whereas John Donne in an earlier century had called childbirth an ominous precipitation, Blake described infants in
positive terms:

> fearless, lustful, happy! nestling for delight
> In laps of pleasure; Innocence! honest, open, seeking
> The vigorous joys of morning light.[2]

People were not born evil but came "trailing clouds of glory
. . . from God, who is our home," to quote Wordsworth
(1770–1850). Sin did not cause disease, pain, and suffering,
as Mather and Wesley had argued. Man sinned only because
the harsh conditions of daily life destroyed his innate purity.
Control poverty, disease, and pain, said the philosophers,
and man would revert to his inherent good behavior. The
high value that society placed on the temporal welfare of
humankind became the basis for the humanitarian movement of the nineteenth century.[3]

The church encouraged the humanitarian movement
and was itself changed by it. People generally became more
aware of cruelty in early Christian schemes of salvation. A
comment by the early nineteenth-century minister and scientist Joseph Priestley illustrates the transition. Though raised
a strict Calvinist, Priestley eventually became a Unitarian.
Before undertaking his ministry in the Unitarian church, he
failed to pass the examination for ordination as a Method-
ist. Priestley said, "When they interrogated me upon the sin
of Adam, I appeared to be not quite orthodox, not thinking
that all the human race were liable to the wrath of God and
the pains of hell forever on account of that sin alone."[4]

Concepts of pain evolved during the eighteenth and

nineteenth centuries, as we can see in the political writings of three English philosophers: John Locke, Jeremy Bentham, and John Stuart Mill. Each wrote extensively about pain and its corollary, pleasure. Each considered pain and pleasure important motives of human behavior, and each built his social philosophy around this point. At the beginning of the eighteenth century pain still had many of its medieval religious connotations. By the end of the nineteenth century pain was conceived as a natural phenomenon and as a destructive, not potentially beneficial, one.

John Locke (1632–1704) believed that pain and pleasure were given by God, a view consistent with traditional interpretations of both the Old and New Testaments. In his definitions of pleasure and pain in *An Essay Concerning Human Understanding* he drew no distinction between the physical and the mental, including "whatsoever delights or molests us; whether it arises from the thoughts of our minds, or anything operating on our bodies." Locke recognized the importance of pain and pleasure as motives for human behavior, noting that nature "put into man a desire of happiness and an aversion to misery . . . which . . . do continue constantly to operate and influence all our actions." He believed that pain, like pleasure, had important functions: "Pain has the same efficacy and use to set us on work that pleasure has. . . . Our Maker, who design[ed] the preservation of our being, has . . . annexed pain to the application of many things to our bodies, to warn us of harm that they will do, and as advices to withdraw from them." He suggested that pain is an adjunct to learning: "Attention and repetition help much to the fixing any ideas in the memory. But those which . . . make the deepest and most lasting impressions, are those which are accompanied with pleasure or pain."[5]

The second philosopher, Jeremy Bentham (1748-1832), was the founder of utilitarianism and one of the most influential theorists of his time. Bentham made pain a central theme of his book *An Introduction to the Principles of Morals and Legislation,* published in 1780 and revised, expanded, and reissued in 1789, 1823, and 1838. Like Locke, Bentham recognized the importance of pleasure and pain as motives of human behavior: "Nature has placed mankind under governance of two sovereign masters, pain and pleasure. It is for them alone to point out what we ought to do as well as to determine what we shall do." He retained the idea that God dispensed pain and pleasure but qualified this by saying that God inflicted pain and awarded pleasure through "natural law" rather than direct intervention. In contrast to Locke, Bentham saw no intrinsic good in pain, calling it "inherently evil." [6]

John Stuart Mill (1806-1873), the most secular of the three philosophers, acknowledged no connection between God and pain in his book *Nature and Utilitarianism.* He attributed pain solely to natural processes, which he thought harsh and capricious. "Nature impales men, breaks them as if on the wheel, casts them to be devoured by wild beasts, burns them to death, crushes them with stones like the first Christian martyr, starves them with hunger, freezes them with cold . . . with the most supercilious disregard both of mercy and justice . . . upon the best and noblest indiferently with the meanest and worst: Even when she does not intend to kill she inflicts the same tortures in apparent wantonness. . . . No human being ever comes into the world but another human being is literally on the rack for hours or days, not infrequently issuing in death." To Mill, the sin of Eve neither explained nor justified the suffering of generations of women. The only value that he allowed to pain and suffering was that they provoked "rational creatures to rise up and struggle against them."[7]

Significantly, none of the three writers mentioned punishment, redemption, and magic, which were traditionally associated with pain. By the early nineteenth century pain and suffering had become secular phenomena, appropriate for study and control by all the methods normally used by scientists.

Biological Perceptions of Pain

Even as political scientists reevaluated the psychological and social significance of pain, physicians and scientists unraveled its biologic properties. The historian Peter Gay believes that a common sense of mission joined philosophers and physicians during the Enlightenment. He suggests that social philosophers saw medicine as a tool to improve life, one that would help lift humans from ignorance and squalor. Physicians, in turn, recognized the potential of new methods of scholarship, using them to study nature and to explore ancient Greek and Arabic medical texts.[8]

The more that scientists studied nature, the more impressed they were by its order. The predictability of natural phenomena proved the existence of God, they said. The study of natural law became, therefore, a form of worship, especially because such work required reason, another of God's gifts. In a book on "haemastaticks," for example, the minister and scientist Stephen Hales described the faith that prompted his original experiments in blood pressure. "There is so just a Symmetry of Parts, such innumerable Beauties and Harmony in the uniform Frame and Texture and of so vast a Variety of solid and fluid Parts, they must ever afford Room for further Discoveries to the diligent Enquirer; and thereby yield fresh instances to illustrate the Wisdom of the divine Architect, the Traces of which are so plain to be seen in every Thing."[9]

In time, however, the study and manipulation of the natural world lost religious overtones; people built factories for economic gain, cultivated art for pleasure, and studied science for its own sake, not simply for the glorification of God. By the end of the eighteenth century, Hume, Voltaire, and other philosophers of the Enlightenment disparaged traditional religious values. They sought to master nature solely for worldly purposes, to "multiply the conveniences or pleasures of life," or, as Descartes said, "to improve health, lengthen life, and banish the terrors of old age." Toward this end, they developed and used new methods for scientific study.[10]

As scientists looked more critically at pain, they refined its meaning. This evolution of thought is apparent even in the works of philosophers and theologians. Early descriptions had been imprecise or scant. Like Locke, few physicians distinguished physical pain from mental suffering. Predictably, neither did Cotton Mather or John Wesley in their medical books. In contrast, Bentham subdivided pain by cause —natural, manmade, or divine. He further identified factors that alter the intensity of pain, such as age, gender, fatigue, and mental condition. The establishment of distinctions, which made pain less mysterious and easier to study, was a necessary first step toward scientific investigation.[11]

Theological connotations of pain changed more as physicians discovered how the body works. Theories of neurological function that dominated medicine at the beginning of the nineteenth century, such as those developed by William Cullen and Benjamin Rush, were vague and fanciful by today's standards, but they did address important questions —How does an organism function? How does it initiate purposeful activity? How does it respond to change in its environment?—which were part of a larger debate concerning the relation between the body and the soul. Some thought the two separate and independent. Others thought them inextricably bound, to the extent that any physical perturbation of the body would affect the soul.[12]

Cullen believed that the nervous system controlled the body by regulating the ebb and flow of energy. He borrowed this idea from Robert Whytt (1714–1766), who preceded him as professor of medicine at Edinburgh. Whytt's ideas, a prominent feature of the medical system taught at Edinburgh, influenced students long after his death. Cullen taught them, and Rush, learning them from Cullen, transported them to the United States.

Whytt realized that individual parts of the body worked together as a unit and thought the nervous system responsible for the coordination. The nervous system derived energy from two sources. The first was innate and varied among individuals depending on age, gender, and disposition— some of the same factors identified by Bentham. The second source consisted of environmental factors, such as living condition, physical exertion, level of education, cultural stimuli, and even pain. Once "sensed," external stimuli either enhanced or diminished the central store of energy. Changes in energy levels induced by the senses initiated appropriate responses.[13]

Whytt's theory explained both voluntary and involuntary behavior. Voluntary behavior began with a spontaneous change in internal energy, whereas involuntary behavior began with stimulation from the environment. Whytt's theory also explained the "particular and very remarkable consent between various parts of the body," by which he meant a coordinated response. "Consent" meant the ability of one organ to respond "in sympathy" to another. "There are only two kinds of motion observed in the bodies of living animals, viz. voluntary, and involuntary from stimuli. In order to effect the performance of the first, the nervous power is not only necessary, but also a free communication, by means of the nerves between the brain, and the parts to be moved." As examples, he mentioned "contraction of the pupil when light offends the eyes, and of the eye-lids when grosser bodies threaten to hurt them." Whytt said, "As many of these complaints depend upon that sympathy which obtains between the various parts of the body, it seemed necessary to begin with some observation on the sympathy of the nerves; a subject of the greatest importance in pathology."[14]

In Whytt's scheme, "sympathy" also described the capacity of one individual to respond to another. The ebb and flow of energy among individuals explained the complex but predictable interactions among members of a social group, just as the ebb and flow of energy within the nervous system explained the complex but coordinated actions of the body.[15]

According to the historian Christopher Lawrence, the social implications of Whytt's theory were particularly important in nineteenth-century Scotland. At the time, social philosophers thought that individuals whose "sensibilities" had been heightened by education and culture not only reacted more to their own pain but also became more "sympathetic" to the pain and suffering of others. The capacity of a social group to respond "in sympathy" was cumulative and formed the basis for a civilized society. Ignorance, hard physical labor, and bad living conditions, on the other hand, made people less sensitive to their own pain and less sympathetic to the pain of others, a combination of factors that destroyed social bonds. Therefore, environmental factors changed society just as it changed individuals. The intelligentsia of Edinburgh believed that their refined sensibilities distinguished them physiologically as well as socially from their compatriots in the Highlands, a group thought to lead rather brutish lives.[16]

Though a simplistic explanation of social behavior, Whytt's theory anticipated biologic concepts that emerged in the nineteenth century. Whytt used "sympathy" and "consent" much as we use such phrases as "nervous reflex" and "integration." When Sir Charles Sherrington received a Nobel Prize in 1932 for demonstrating that complex animal behavior could be analyzed as if it were a collection of reflexes coordinated to achieve a specific goal, he simply solved a biologic problem that Whytt had described years before.[17] Whytt's idea that external stimuli permanently alter the nervous system has credence in modern science. Examples of such phenomena include the behavioral imprinting of newborn animals, the "cortical blindness" of animals deprived of light from birth, and the increased verbal skills of people exposed to foreign languages during infancy. Considering the limits of science in the eighteenth century, Whytt did quite well.

An important movement away from Whytt's explanation of nervous function emerged in 1811, when Sir Charles Bell and François Magendie suggested that the dorsal and ventral roots of the spinal cord have different functions, a theory soon substantiated experimentally by Magendie. Shortly thereafter, J. J. Legallois discovered a discrete area in the lower portion of the brain that controls respiration (1812), Pierre Flourens identified the cerebellum as the portion of the brain that coordinates body movements (1824), and the great German physiologist Johannes Müller announced his doctrine of specific nerve energy. According to Müller, the body has special sensors for different stimuli—for pressure, say, temperature, and touch. Regardless of the nature of the activating stimulus, a given kind of receptor will produce only one kind of sensation. Any sensation produced by a receptor specialized to sense pressure would be perceived as pressure even if the receptor was activated by an electric current.

Meanwhile, clinical work by some English physicians and innumerable French physicians demonstrated the relation between lesions in specific areas of the brain and recognizable clinical disorders. The suggestion that pain, too, was mediated by discrete pathways was made in 1846, the year of Morton's anesthetic triumph.

These discoveries altered concepts of nervous function. No longer were internal and external stimuli considered to merely augment or diminish an amorphous pool of nervous energy. Rather, stimuli excited anatomically discrete receptors, each of which initiated an electrical impulse that traveled along a specific nerve to a localized area of the brain. The brain interpreted the signal, integrating it with signals received from other parts of the body, and initiated an appropriate response.

For scientists and physicians, such discoveries made pain a process that they could manipulate. Surgery could destroy receptors, interrupt nerve pathways, or extirpate areas of the brain responsible for interpreting signals or initiating responses. The possibility of manipulating the pain process with chemicals, such as ether or chloroform, probably seemed quite reasonable. News of such studies helped prepare the public for Simpson's work.[18]

Sensitivity to the Pain of Childbirth

One aspect of Whytt's theory—that education and culture permanently altered both the structure and function of the nervous system—continued to have credence. For J. S. Jewell, a widely quoted American physician, it accounted for the rising incidence of mental illness. "There can be no question as to whether the nervous systems of highly cultivated and refined individuals among civilized peoples are more complex and refined in structure and delicate in susceptibility and action, at least in their higher parts, than the nervous systems of savages." According to the theory, one sensibility that remained undeveloped in savages was the "sensitivity" to pain. "In our process of being civilized we have won . . . [an] intensified capacity to suffer," wrote Silas Wier Mitchell, an another American physician, in 1892. "The savage does not feel pain as we do." On this premise, the privileged class reasoned that it needed anesthesia more than other classes.[19]

Physicians and the public applied the same argument to childbirth. Lacking sensibility, animals do not experience labor pain, they said; savages and lower-class women experience less labor pain than women who are educated and cultured. Thus, the obstetrician Thomas Denman wrote that "lower orders of women have more easy and favorable births, than those who live in affluence . . . they suffer less because they are stronger, and have less feeling and apprehension." George Engelmann was even more explicit in a book, *Labor Among Primitive Peoples,* written eight decades later (1882):

> Among primitive people, still natural in their habits and living under conditions which favor the healthy development of their physical organization, labor may be characterized as short and easy, accompanied by few accidents and followed by little or no prostrations. . . . The nearer civilization is approached, the more trying does the ordeal of childbirth [become]. . . . The system suffers from the abuses of civilization, its dissipations, and the follies of fashion. On account of the idle life led, and the relaxed condition of the uterus and abdominal walls, there is a greater tendency to malpositions; additional difficulties are presented by the weakened organization, and the languid neurasthenic conditions of the subjects in civilized communities.

The suffragette Elizabeth Cady Stanton agreed. "Refined, genteel, civilized women have worse labor pain." After her own almost painless delivery she remarked "Am I not almost a savage?"[20]

Simpson rejected this thesis. He said that all women in labor suffer equally and that women experience more pain than animals, not because of cultural factors but because structural changes in the pelvis associated with an upright posture required a thicker, more powerful uterus to expel the child.

Engelmann's book added an interesting twist to earlier concepts of pain. Whereas Whytt had thought increased sensitivity to pain a mark of education and civility, Engelmann called it evidence of deterioration, a loss of inherent strength and wisdom on the part of those who had once lived in a more natural state. These opinions probably reflected differences in social prejudices. Whytt had been a member of the upper class in a country that was proud of the cultural differences that distinguished one social class from another. Engelmann lived in the United States toward the end of the era of Jacksonian democracy, in which the public decried class distinctions and extolled the virtues of the "noble savage," described in the romantic and very popular novels of James Fenimore Cooper.

In spite of its popularity, Engelmann's book contained little of scientific substance: no data, no estimates of the severity of childbirth pain, no measurements of the duration of labor, no comparisons of the frequency of medical complications between groups of "civilized" and "savage" women. The book consisted simply of anecdotes describing childbirth practices in different cultures, collected from various sources. Presumably, it became popular because it confirmed prevailing beliefs. Similar ideas can be found as late as 1933 in the arguments that Grantly Dick Read used to establish his method of "natural childbirth."[21]

An Era of Optimism and Reform

Throughout the first half of the nineteenth century western Europeans and Americans wanted thoroughgoing reforms and were willing to sacrifice to instate them. Between 1776 and 1850 they put into practice many of the ideas developed during the Renaissance and the Enlightenment. Great changes occurred: four major political upheavals (the American, French, and German revolutions and the Napoleonic

Wars); an industrial revolution and agrarian reform; and important advances in physics, geology (Lyell), biology (the cell theory of Schleiden and Schwann), and chemistry (Lavoisier, Priestley, and Scheele). Within twenty years after the invention of the steam locomotive in 1827, almost seven thousand miles of track were laid in Great Britain alone.

In the British Empire, Victoria's coronation in 1837 ushered in a period of prosperity and expansion. In the United States, Andrew Jackson's inauguration as president, though depressing to intellectuals, marked a surge of populism, a movement that had repercussions for science and medicine. Americans rode a wave of optimism generated by their great political experiment, by their recovery from the economic depression of 1837–1842, by the western migration, spurred in part by the discovery of gold at Sutter's Mill in 1848, and access to the untapped resources of the continent—the Louisiana Purchase had doubled the area of the country in 1803—and by a sense of self-reliance, fostered, as suggested by the historian Frederick Jackson Turner, by the experience of dealing with the isolation of wilderness life. Western Europeans and Americans were suffused with extraordinary energy and a sense of boundless progress. Not only had they transformed their outlook on the world, but they found both the resolve and the means to change the structure and function of many social institutions. Francis Bacon's early comment, "Man is the architect of his fortune," captured the mood of the era.[22] Developments in medicine kept pace with these other improvements.

It would be naive to oversimplify the motivation for humanitarianism, a movement so diverse that it embraced labor and child welfare reform, women's suffrage, welfare programs for the poor, reform of prisons and schools, antivivisectionism, and the abolition of slavery.[23] Common to all these social programs, however, was the preoccupation with pain and suffering described by William James in 1901. Public inquiries into atrocious working conditions, including the physical abuse of women and children in mines and factories, led to work reform. Publicity surrounding experiments on unanesthetized animals, even those by such prominent scientists as Magendie and Bernard, stoked the antivivisection movement. News reports including graphic descriptions of blood sports won support for newly formed societies for the protection of animals. Publicity about deaths of soldiers from floggings led to reform of military discipline in England, just as revelations about hazing and brutal discipline prompted Thomas Arnold's reform of British public schools.

In short, abolition of pain and suffering became a major motive for reform of nineteenth-century society. Early in the movement Thomas Jefferson changed Locke's phrase "life, liberty, and estate" to "life, liberty, and the pursuit of happiness," a transformation that epitomized the emphasis now placed on happiness—which could be defined as freedom from pain. This is not to say that needless cruelty suddenly disappeared from Western society. After the Enlightenment, however, western Europeans and Americans began a prolonged effort to eliminate suffering from human experience, a tendency that was not particularly apparent before then.

Early advocates of anesthesia were part of this great humanitarian movement. John Snow; his close friend and biographer, Benjamin Ward Richardson; and John Collins Warren, the surgeon who performed the surgery on the patient whom Morton anesthetized, were prominent in the animal rights movement in the first part of the century. Walter Channing and his brother, the Unitarian minister William Ellery Channing, were close to several New England abolitionists. Simpson himself had strong humanitarian sentiments: "The true moral question is, 'Is a practitioner justified by any principles of humanity in not using it [anesthesia]?' I believe every operation without it is just a piece of the most deliberate and cold-blooded cruelty."[24]

The acceptance of anesthesia came during a period of social change and political activism. The ability of anesthesia to obliterate pain dramatized the ability of science to overcome the dark forces of nature and to improve life on earth. It epitomized the spirit of the Enlightenment and justified widespread optimism. John Stuart Mill predicted that "most of the great positive evils of the world are . . . removable and . . . will be in the end completely extinguished by the wisdom of society . . . even the most intractable of enemies, disease." Edward H. Clarke, a professor at Harvard, observed, "Anesthetic agents . . . enabled the physician at his will to compel pain to disappear and distress to be quiet." Public repudiation of childbirth pain was also a manifestation of this philosophy. Oliver Wendell Holmes, professor of anatomy at Harvard, said: "The agony which seemed inseparable from maternity has been divorced from it, in the face of the ancestral curse resting upon woman-hood. With the first painless birth, induced by an anesthetic agent, the reign of tradition was over, and humanity was ready to assert all its rights."[25] To nations that set out to explore and change the whole world, the alleviation of the pain of childbirth must have seemed a rather trivial technical problem. In another social environment, however, it seems unlikely that Morton and Simpson would have enjoyed the success that they did.

Shortly after Simpson introduced obstetric anesthesia, he predicted that patients "would force its use upon the profession." This proved to be the case. Reflecting the general spirit of the age, women were enthusiastic. Queen Victoria, after receiving her first anesthetic for childbirth, spoke of "this blessed chloroform." When her oldest daughter, Vickey, delivered her first child in 1859, the queen remarked, "What a blessing she had chloroform. Without it I think her strength would have suffered very much." [26]

Physicians were timid about using anesthesia on the queen and not ready to agree to administer anesthesia to Fanny Longfellow, a pioneer user in the United States. Finding courageous physicians was difficult at first. Fanny Longfellow's courage and enthusiasm convinced friends to try the innovation, but they, too, had difficulty finding compliant physicians. Some women without medical recourse had their husbands administer the anesthesia. In 1856 one Massachusetts physician remarked that once he had administered anesthesia to a patient, "in every case, if I am called to a succeeding labor, the first question has invariably been 'Have you brought the chloroform?'" [27]

In time, physicians did become more comfortable giving anesthesia to patients in labor. According to textbooks published during the last decades of the nineteenth century, any physician practicing obstetrics had to have that skill. Trying to find something better than ether and chloroform, physicians experimented with new drugs, but except for nitrous oxide, the "laughing gas" from earlier in the century, few lasted.

Public pressure notwithstanding, most physicians remained cautious about obstetric anesthesia. Although they recommended using anesthesia in the management of spe-

cial obstetric problems—for example, surgical deliveries and
eclampsia—they continued to discourage its use for normal labor. In an extensive survey conducted in 1875, most
of the four hundred physicians who responded expressed
the same medical concerns as obstetricians of the preceding
generation.[28]

Physicians had reason for concern. By 1900 there had
been several studies of deaths during anesthesia. Zweifel had
demonstrated that drugs do cross the placenta, and other
physicians had reason to believe that the newborn was especially sensitive. Physicians had not resolved the question of
the effects of anesthesia on uterine contractions. One prominent obstetrician suggested anesthesia increased the risk of
puerperal fever. Those who recommended anesthesia suggested limiting the amount given and restricting its use to
the actual time of delivery. They emphasized that administration was an "art to be acquired."[29]

Some resistance to anesthesia even developed in Simpson's home city of Edinburgh. One physician, J. Mathews
Duncan, noted that "anesthesia is not so much used now
as it was, and much less freely when it is employed. It is
fashionable to have chloroform, and often the use of it is a
mere farce in deference to fashion. The fashion was fostered
by exaggerated pictures being drawn of the pains of natural labour." True or not, patients were no longer prepared
to accept pain when they believed that their physicians had
effective methods to relieve it.[30]

In the course of time, patients and physicians developed
divergent views about obstetric anesthesia. Women wanted
no pain, and those with money or influence found ways to
have anesthesia. Physicians, who were dealing with issues of
safety and medicine, remained concerned and cautious. As

the gap between the views of patients and physicians on the issue of "Twilight Sleep" widened in the first decades of the twentieth century, particularly in the United States, the debate became public and acrimonious.

CHAPTER EIGHT

"There Ought to Be No Pain"

The American Women's Campaign for Twilight Sleep

All she asked was that nothing should "hurt" her: she had the

blind dread of physical pain common also to most of the young

women of her set. But all that was so easily managed nowadays:

Mrs. Manford . . . of course knew the most perfect "Twilight

Sleep" establishment in the country, installed Lita in its most

luxurious suite, and filled her rooms with its spring flowers,

hot-house fruits, new novels and all the latest picture-papers —

and Lita drifted into motherhood as lightly and unperceivingly

as if the wax doll which suddenly appeared in the cradle at her bedside had been brought there in one of the big bunches of

hot-house roses that she found every morning on her pillow.

"Of course there ought to be no Pain . . . nothing but Beauty.

. . . It ought to be one of the loveliest, most poetic things in the

world to have a baby," Mrs. Manford declared, in that bright

efficient voice which made liveliness and poetry sound like

the attributes of an advanced industrialism, and babies

something to be turned out in series, like Fords.

—Edith Wharton, *Twilight Sleep,* 1927

The convictions that prompted so many social reforms during the first half of the nineteenth century continued during the last half but took some new directions, eventually affecting even the use of anesthesia for childbirth. Feminist issues became more prominent after 1848, the year of the Seneca Falls Convention, from which many mark the beginning of the women's suffrage movement in America. At first, American women campaigned for the right to vote and for improvements in their economic, legal, and social status. By the turn of the century they had become increasingly concerned with women's health and childbirth. Abhorrence of pain and suffering continued to be an important impetus for social change.

Physicians may have admired the idealism that prompted social reform, but such idealism did not affect their practice of medicine. Still influenced by the skepticism that had freed them from Galenic medicine, physicians continued to discuss, test, and criticize every new idea before accepting change. Of this period the medical historian Richard Shryock has observed, "When such apostles of German thought as Coleridge, Carlyle, and Emerson sought to convert the English-speaking peoples, it was largely the religious leaders or the artistically minded who responded. Medical workers proved indifferent, or regarded the idealists with cold and quizzical eyes. . . . Poets might lament the pathos of early death, but to French and Austrian clinicians . . . death was but a scientific fact."[1]

The social idealism of American feminists finally collided with the analytic methods of physicians in 1914, when women learned of a new way to manage the pain of labor. Its German innovators called it *Dämmerschlaf,* or Twilight Sleep. Women hailed Twilight Sleep as a triumph of tech-

nology. Physicians, in contrast, viewed it with "cold and quizzical eyes" and began their tedious process of discussion
and clinical study. Frustrated by the delay and perceiving
delay as disinterest, American women confronted physicians
in a battle that pitched their social goals against twentieth-
century methods of medical science.

Twilight Sleep in Germany

The anesthetic method of Twilight Sleep was not entirely
new. Surgeons had used it since 1900. By 1907 an Austrian
physician, Richard von Steinbüchel, had adapted it for obstetrics. Shortly thereafter, acceptance of the method gained
momentum when two German obstetricians from Freiburg,
Carl Gauss and Bernhardt Krönig, modified and publicized
the technique. By 1914 Twilight Sleep was used in several
prominent European hospitals.[2]

Twilight Sleep combined morphine and scopolamine,
two drugs that physicians knew quite well. For centuries
morphine and its parent compound, opium, had been used
to treat pain and many other medical problems, ones as
dissimilar as venereal disease and psychosis. Scopolamine,
another plant extract, was known to be a poison capable
of causing confusion, disorientation, and amnesia. Hamlet's
father is murdered with henbane, a source of scopolamine.
Unlike ether and chloroform, which produce a state of anesthesia—that is, complete freedom from pain and total unconsciousness—Twilight Sleep offered analgesia, or partial pain
relief, and amnesia.

Used separately, morphine and scopolamine had serious limitations in obstetrics. Most experts believed that the
amount of morphine needed to abolish the pain of labor
would depress the mother's uterine contractions and the

newborn's respiration. Scopolamine did induce amnesia and sleep, two advantages, but it also caused urinary retention and an unpleasantly dry mouth and made many patients delirious, hallucinatory, and physically difficult to control. Gauss believed he could gain the benefit of each drug without incurring its risks if he gave the drugs together but in smaller amounts.

Because Gauss recognized the thin margin between the therapeutic and toxic effects of Twilight Sleep, his instructions for its use were precise. The first injection, given shortly after the start of active labor, was to consist of simultaneous administration of both drugs. The small amount of morphine contained in the injection—ten milligrams—was all the patient would receive for the entire labor. For most patients, this dose of morphine blunted but did not eliminate all the pain. After the initial injection of both drugs, patients received only scopolamine, its dose adjusted to obliterate the memory of labor.

Choosing the right amount of scopolamine required judgment. Too much was toxic. Too little left "islands of memory" or, worse yet, recall of the entire period of labor. Women wanted amnesia so that they, like the heroine in Edith Wharton's novel, could drift into "motherhood as lightly and unperceivingly" as possible. To circumvent the risk of recall, Gauss devised a memory test. During labor he asked patients simple questions and had them perform simple tasks. Only if they responded correctly did he administer more scopolamine.

Even with careful adjustment of the dose, many patients became confused and disoriented with Twilight Sleep. Freed of their inhibitions by scopolamine but still in pain, they screamed and thrashed about. Gauss found that he could minimize this reaction by eliminating extraneous "sensory input." He kept his patients in a dark and quiet room, bandaged their eyes with gauze, and stuffed their ears with wads of cotton soaked in oil. To prevent patients from injuring themselves, Gauss confined them to a padded bed and kept an attendant or a physician constantly by their side. During delivery of the child he often restrained a patient's arms with leather thongs and supplemented Twilight Sleep with a general anesthetic. Like the heroine in Edith Wharton's novel, most of Gauss's patients remembered nothing of the labor, the delivery, or the hours immediately thereafter, and they sometimes even forgot the following days.

The American Campaign

The public, no less than physicians, recognized the limitations of ether and chloroform for childbirth. Although Simpson and Channing asserted the contrary, anesthesia was known to slow labor. Ether made patients sick, and chloroform could destroy the liver. Sudden and unexpected death had occurred often enough during chloroform anesthesia to warrant study by a special commission (in India). Safe administration of either drug required experienced and skilled people, few of whom were available. Physicians had sought substitute drugs, but all experiments had failed. Most women delivered babies as they had for centuries, in pain and without medical relief.[3] The public was ready for something new, especially a technique developed by Germans; many acknowledged German medicine as the best in the world. When Twilight Sleep came along, many people thought it the ideal solution for the problems of childbirth.

Intense interest in Twilight Sleep developed among a small group of wealthy American women who heard of it and went to Germany to try it. One early enthusiast was

Mrs. C. Temple Emmet, a granddaughter of the Astors. She traveled to Freiburg for delivery of each of her three children. In 1914 *McClure's Magazine* sent two journalists, Mary Boyd and Marguerite Tracy, to Germany to gather material for a special story. While there, Boyd delivered her own child under Gauss's care. Tracy and another American, Constance Leupp, described the method in a long article that appeared in *McClure's* later that year.[4] According to the authors and the editors, the article evoked more response from readers than any other that the magazine had ever published.

Tracy and Leupp featured in their article personal comments from Boyd about her own delivery and studio pictures of Gauss and many "Freiburg Babies"—well-dressed, attractive children whose mothers had received Twilight Sleep for their deliveries. The article also included long quotations from the director of the Freiburg Frauenklinik, Bernhardt Krönig, an aggressive young professor already known for challenging the dominance of Berlin academics and for finding gynecologic applications for radiography, a new diagnostic tool.

Krönig was quoted on the need for better ways to relieve the pain of childbirth. He described the permanent debilitating effects of severe pain and the susceptibility of "mothers of the better classes" to pain and other obstetrical problems. In a statement reminiscent of Robert Whytt's eighteenth-century views, Krönig cited environmental factors as causing changes in the physical responses of the nervous system. "The modern woman, on whose nervous system nowadays quite other demands are made than was formerly the case, responds to the stimulus of severe pain more rapidly with nervous exhaustion and paralysis of the will . . . the sensitiveness of those who carry on hard mental work is greater than that of those who earn their living by manual labor."

Greater susceptibility to pain made such women more need-
ful of relief, he said, and Twilight Sleep offered that relief
in a completely safe, highly effective way. The article stimulated interest among women of other social classes, not just
the monied ones.

In the garden of the Frauenklinik several American
women recuperating from childbirth discussed their satisfaction with Twilight Sleep. From this conversation in 1914 arose
the idea of the National Twilight Sleep Association, an organization dedicated to publicizing the method and increasing
its use in the United States. Mrs. C. Temple Emmet became
president. Another Freiburg mother, Mrs. Cecil Stewart, the
sister of Marguerite Tracy, became secretary. Others who
served on the original board included several women prominent in New York social circles, among them an author, an
actress, and the wife of the U.S. commissioner for immi-
gration.

The goals, structure, and methods of the National Twilight Sleep Association were similar to those of many organizations active at that time. After the Civil War, women formed
many groups to improve the social, political, and legal status
of women and children. As women became more concerned
with health issues later in the century, they founded hospitals and clinics to train nurses and women physicians and to
improve medical care for indigent mothers and children. Examples are the New England Women's Medical Society, the
Visiting Nurse Service of the City of New York, the New York
Nursery and Child's Hospital, and the New England Hospital for Women and Children.[5]

The rationale for this early feminist movement was
complex. Underlying much of its work was the conviction
that women would have better opportunities only if they
themselves campaigned for change. Reformers assumed that

women, by both nature and experience, were more "sensitive" (as the word was used by Whytt and Hume) than men to the physical and mental suffering of others. This quality made them better prepared to change the conditions responsible for suffering. Although feminist organizations drew most of their support from women of the upper class, they worked to improve the status of all.

The ideology that sparked the early feminist movement also ignited the campaigns for Twilight Sleep and for improvements in obstetrical care. As one obstetrician observed:

> On the surface of the Woman's Movement floats the great vessel known as the Vote . . . there is underneath . . . a deep ground swell of discontent — in many cases well founded — of dissatisfaction with the life of womankind under certain circumstances and of actual rebellion against the imposed self-sacrifice of the mother's lot. . . . Now, if we obstetricians, who have by anaesthetics taken the sting out of labour and its pain, can by hygiene, supervision, and treatment remove some at least of the irksomeness from the nine months of pregnancy and the whole of the danger, we shall have done much to solve a part and not an inconsiderable part of the women's question.[6]

To Tracy and Boyd, also, Twilight Sleep was an important part of the feminist movement. "American women of today believe that the weariness, the physiological depression, the disturbance of function, the giving out of nourishment and energy, the loss of good looks, the withdrawal from the customary resources of social life in pregnancy are enough of a sacrifice to the future. . . . Not a few women of good normal minds have gone to seed, become dumb, patient, brooding animals after the exhaustion of a succession of painful births." They also noted how the "tortures and miseries of childbirth" prompted American women to demand "that medical science shall create the environment and fulfil the exacting requirements for . . . Twilight Sleep." They suggested that the campaign for Twilight Sleep signified "the first time in the history of medical science that the whole body of patients has risen to dictate to the doctors." The outcome of the struggle would "relieve one-half of humanity from its antique burden of a suffering which the other half of humanity has never understood."[7]

A comment by another advocate of Twilight Sleep also illustrates the connection between the medical management of the pain of childbirth and the goals of feminists: "The insistence of the American women that they shall have the benefits of the new method is bringing results. Keep on ladies! Hammer away with all your might. Emancipation day has come."[8]

The campaign for Twilight Sleep began in 1914 shortly after popular support for other women's issues had increased. The campaign for women's education in the nineteenth century had led to the foundation of many new women's colleges.[9] In the early twentieth century more women went on to advanced studies after college than ever before. The long campaign for women's suffrage moved closer to success: five years after the formation of the National Twilight Sleep Association, the U.S. Congress ratified the amendment that gave women the right to vote. Leaders of the National Twilight Sleep Association had close ties with other feminist organizations, and several of its board members were active in the campaign for women's suffrage. Eight of the twenty board members were listed in the *Who's Who Among Ameri-*

can Women for 1914–1915. Given its mission and political connections, the association quickly won endorsement by the prestigious New York Federation of Women's Clubs. From within medicine, support for Twilight Sleep came from only a handful of physicians, among them W. H. Wellington Knipe, an obstetrician practicing at Gouvenour's Hospital in New York. In a nicely balanced article published in 1914, Knipe reviewed existing literature and concluded that Twilight Sleep held great promise.[10] Lay proponents of the method cited his opinion often. Among physicians, however, Knipe was an exception.

The National Twilight Sleep Association launched an extensive and aggressive campaign to counteract physicians' resistance. It published pamphlets, arranged lectures, and staged rallies in department stores in northeastern cities. Within a year Tracy, Leupp, and Boyd had published a book and two additional articles dealing with Twilight Sleep. Other authors published supportive articles in the *Literary Digest,* the *Ladies' Home Journal,* and the *Reader's Digest* and in an assortment of books for public consumption.[11]

As public interest increased, more physicians used Twilight Sleep for their patients. Dr. Bertha van Hoosen, an advocate even before the *McClure's* article, established a special obstetric unit in Chicago. Similar units appeared in Boston, New York, and even Brooklyn, the last through the work of Mrs. Francis X. Carmody, another Freiburg mother and an active member of the National Twilight Sleep Association. Twilight Sleep even gained support from editors of the *New York Times.* During a fifteen-month period more than a dozen stories and editorials appeared in its pages praising the method and criticizing physicians who opposed it.[12]

Lay articles promoting Twilight Sleep shared several characteristics. Their authors endorsed the assertion that the process of civilization had caused the physical deterioration of women and had made them more sensitive to the debilitating effects of pain. They described childbirth as "torture" and suggested that the prospect of pain deterred many women from becoming pregnant, particularly upper-class and better-educated women, who, they said, should be the ones to have the largest families. The writer of one book described a pregnant woman driven to suicide by her fear of the impending pain of childbirth.

In articles and editorials alike American physicians were accused of rejecting Twilight Sleep because of its promotion by patients rather than medical colleagues, because of procrastination in learning about the subject, or a callous indifference to the pain of women in labor. Had doctors "thought less of their own convenience and interests and more of sparing women pain always agonizing and perils often fatal, [they] could long since have freed childbirth of its terrors and lifted the 'primal curse.'" Proponents of Twilight Sleep said that physicians had rejected the method without serious consideration, much as they had rejected other major medical ideas, such as the development of vaccination to prevent smallpox and the contagious nature of puerperal fever. "In short, 'medical authority' was unanimous against the 'twilight sleep' just as it had been a hundred times before against changes in practice afterward accepted as of priceless value." The press and authors of popular books, criticizing the medical reports describing complications of Twilight Sleep, also argued that the method was safe and would work well if only physicians would adhere to the original guidelines of Gauss.[13]

Unfortunately, material in the lay press contained remarkably little detail about patients' reactions to pain when they were treated with Twilight Sleep, which meant that the public received a biased view. No popular articles or books mentioned how patients screamed or thrashed in pain. None described the blindfolds, earplugs, and restraints that Gauss used to control his patients. None included comments from a paper delivered by Krönig at the Clinical Congress of Surgeons of North America in which he described how Twilight Sleep may diminish uterine contractions, depress the onset of respiration in newborns, and cause such "confusion of mind and excitement" that visitors were required to leave the patient for the duration of the labor lest it "make an unpleasant impression." [14] With few exceptions, lay writers relied on information provided by physicians, like Gauss and Krönig, who had developed the method, or the accounts of former patients, like Mary Boyd, who had no memory of labor and delivery. Accordingly, the articles implied that women drifted to sleep after the first injection and awakened refreshed twelve to twenty-four hours later, having delivered a strong, healthy, and intelligent child.

There were disclaimers. Three months after the original story by Tracy and Leupp, the *New York Times* published a long article by an American physician who had observed Twilight Sleep while pursuing medical studies in Europe. Unfortunately, the headline, "Twilight Sleep Is Successful in 120 Cases Here," belied its sobering content. The author described patients who had experienced, and remembered experiencing, great pain. He also mentioned that many German hospitals had already abandoned Twilight Sleep, finding it ineffective and costly. Another American physician who had also worked in Germany corroborated the content of the article in a letter written to the *New York Times*. Even Gauss's original article had sounded notes of caution. He had described the great care necessary in the preparation of the drugs, the need for conservative doses, the special attendants required to protect patients, and the frequency of failures.[15] But none of these publications diminished the enthusiasm that editors and journalists of the *New York Times* or the officers of the National Twilight Sleep Association had for Twilight Sleep.

Physicians' Objections

Contrary to editorials in the *New York Times* and to the opinions of many patients, physicians had considered the value of Twilight Sleep. An influential professor of obstetrics from Johns Hopkins, J. Whitridge Williams, had mentioned the method in two early editions of his textbook, each published several years before the founding of the National Twilight Sleep Association. Williams had warned of problems and had found Twilight Sleep not "suitable for private practice." Joseph DeLee, a Chicago obstetrician no less influential than Williams, made a special trip to Freiburg to observe Twilight Sleep. He, too, was unimpressed, having noted "unsatisfactory results in 10 of 10 cases." In November 1914, American physicians who had given Twilight Sleep to patients met at the New York Academy of Medicine to discuss the method. After a presentation by A. M. Hellman entitled "A New Method of Painless Childbirth," seventeen obstetricians spoke. Some liked Twilight Sleep, but others described complications, such as newborn apnea (failure to breath), inadequate analgesia, unexpected fetal death, and serious postpartum hemorrhage—some of the same problems mentioned a year earlier by Krönig.[16]

As medical debate continued, it focused on three issues: Does Twilight Sleep slow or stop labor? Does it interfere with the respiration of the newborn? Does it work well enough to justify the risks? Before American physicians had direct experience with Twilight Sleep, they used their own clinical experience with opioids to answer these questions, and their fear of Twilight Sleep for childbirth came in part from their knowledge of the effects of opioids given for other medical conditions. For years physicians had used opioids for "colic," a general medical term describing painful abdominal cramps associated with a variety of conditions, such as diarrhea, kidney stones, and gall bladder attacks. Opioids were effective because they not only relieved pain but also slowed or stopped pain-producing contractions of smooth muscle (specialized muscle found in the wall of abdominal organs, such as the gastrointestinal tract, urinary bladder, gall bladder, and uterus). For many medical conditions, physicians had used opioids expressly to stop such contractions. Deaths from cholera, for example, were often related to the loss of body salt and fluids because of diarrhea. Administration of opioids slowed or stopped spasms of the gastrointestinal tract and thus increased survival from cholera. In other circumstances, the same property of opioids caused problems. Used to treat toothache pain, opioids could cause severe urinary retention or constipation.[17]

Obstetricians knew that opioids could relieve the pain of labor, but they feared that opioids would also stop contractions of the uterus. In fact, experts often recommended opioids for just that purpose—to stop premature labor, to provide an interval of rest during a long or severe labor, to stop contractions so that the child could be turned in utero, or to stop contractions in those rare circumstances in which the uterus ruptured during labor. Because of these experiences, they reasoned that opioids would be dangerous to use when continuous contractions were needed during a normal labor or when strong, sustained contractions were needed postpartum to staunch the flow of blood from the placental bed.[18]

When Gauss suggested using morphine as part of his regimen for Twilight Sleep, he was challenging the well-established medical dictum that opioids stop labor. He was also reviving a medical controversy that had lain dormant since 1847. Simpson's contention that uterine pain and uterine contractions were distinct and unrelated had never been proven. Twilight Sleep forced physicians to readdress an issue that they had ignored for almost half a century, this time in regard to opioids rather than ether or chloroform.

Medical science was more sophisticated in 1914 than in Simpson's day. Through the work of French, German, and English medical scientists, physicians knew more about normal and pathologic body functions. With regard to the effects of morphine on labor, medical theory gave extra reason for concern. Throughout the nineteenth century, physiologists had taught that the brain controlled all vital body functions. By 1914 physiologists knew a great deal about respiration, the nuclei in the base of the brain that control respiration, the character of neurologic reflexes that interact with the nuclei, and the environmental stimuli that alter respiration through their effects on the nervous system.[19] Theories about the neural regulation of respiration were extrapolated to other bodily processes, such as parturition.

Physiologists believed that the nervous system controlled labor, just as it controlled respiration. One, W. H. Howell, a colleague of Williams's at Johns Hopkins, taught this principle, and so did Michael Foster of Cambridge University, founder of one of the most influential schools of physiology of that era. In a textbook Foster wrote, "The whole process of parturition may be broadly considered as a reflex act." Obstetricians concurred. Textbooks published earlier in the century attributed the control of labor to the nervous system. Fifty years later Williams's textbook contained similar material, even to the point of including experimental data, an unusual addition for a medical book at that time.[20]

Influenced perhaps by his Johns Hopkins colleague, Williams described the role of brain nuclei in the control of labor. He also mentioned how suckling and dilation of the vagina initiate reflex—that is, involuntary—uterine contractions, a phenomenon well known to practicing physicians, and speculated that anemia and stress may initiate premature labor by stimulating the nuclei in question. He warned, however, that opioids, ether, and chloroform slow or stop labor by depressing the center that normally controls labor. Physicians were ready to accept this warning. Pharmacologists had already shown that opioids, ether, and chloroform were able to depress all components of the nervous system to the point of suspending spontaneous respiration and contractions of the heart, thus causing death.[21]

Physicians were far more concerned about the effect of opioids on labor than they need have been. We now know that the nervous system has a much smaller effect on uterine contractions than was previously thought. In 1914 the clinical and experimental evidence necessary for a change in theory had just begun to accumulate. Physicians knew of women who had had successful labors despite severe spinal cord damage. German scientists had shown that animals could conceive, carry a pregnancy to term, and deliver following a normal labor even after complete surgical destruction of the spinal cord. The introduction of spinal anesthesia to obstetrics in 1903 raised doubts because it became apparent that labor progressed normally even after the uterus had been denervated pharmacologically.[22]

Regardless of the evidence, physicians clung to their old theory of the neurologic control of labor. At first they tried to modify traditional theory to make it consistent with the new data. Instead of attributing the control of labor to a single nucleus in the lower portion of the brain, physicians postulated a second regulatory center in the spinal cord, one capable of functioning independently in the event of spinal cord damage elsewhere. When subsequent observations made this theory untenable, they speculated that nerves "intrinsic to the uterus" might serve the same purpose.[23]

The discovery that finally allowed physicians to develop a theory that would accommodate all the facts was still several years away from the debate about Twilight Sleep. Hormonal regulation, a control mechanism related to but independent of the nervous system, had yet to be discovered. The English physiologist E. H. Starling did not coin the term *hormone* until 1905, and thirty years would pass before anyone isolated estrogen, progesterone, oxytocin, or prostaglandins, much less showed their role in the initiation and regulation of labor. Only recently have physiologists begun to unravel the complex interaction between neural and endocrine regulation of pregnancy.

Some nineteenth-century physicians challenged the idea that opioids stop labor. In 1869 a New Jersey obstetrician suggested that opioids stimulate the nervous system and, therefore, facilitate labor. His comment reflected the uncertainty that had existed among pharmacologists earlier in the century, who could not decide whether opioids stimulated rather than depressed the central nervous system. Although the issue had never been resolved, most physicians agreed with Williams that opioids act primarily as depressants. Experiments by a German obstetrician raised more doubts.[24] He placed special balloons in the uterine cavity to measure the strength of contractions of laboring women before and after administration of morphine. He observed no effect, but most physicians overlooked his data, so they had no discernible impact on medical theory or practice.

In 1914 most physicians still believed that pain and contractions were inextricably joined. Most obstetricians agreed with William Tyler-Smith, the early opponent of obstetric anesthesia who said, "In the present state of our knowledge upon this point, no practitioner can use opium with decision and satisfaction."[25] Because clinical experience and medical theory gave ample reason for caution, Gauss was wise to recommend small amounts of morphine, and obstetricians were right to challenge even that recommendation.

The second focus of the medical debate over Twilight Sleep, after concern for its effects on labor, was concern for the neonate. Although Zweifel's experiments in 1876 had left no doubt that drugs could cross the placenta, physicians seemed unsure how to use the information. By 1914 there were more reports of fetuses dying unexpectedly after administration of opioids to the mother and of neonates failing to breathe. In textbooks and clinical papers warnings appeared that newborns might be more sensitive to opioids than older children or adults. As early as 1842, one pharmacologist said, "In nursing mothers, morphine is apt to be excreted in the milk and will narcotize the child . . . children in utero are also influenced. In all these instances care is necessary."[26]

Initial descriptions of Twilight Sleep did not allay early fears. Despite using small doses of morphine, as recommended by Gauss, obstetricians reported problems. DeLee, for one, cited neonatal "narcosis and asphyxia" among the complications that he had observed during his special trip to the Freiburg clinic. Another obstetrician, B. Cook-Hirst, described a similar experience in Freiburg. Pharmacology textbooks sounded the same alarm. Eventually investigators showed that the doses of morphine that Gauss had recommended were relatively safe and were unlikely to harm the child. But in 1914 physicians still did not know that.[27]

The third issue that dogged medical investigators was the efficacy of Twilight Sleep. Anyone who had observed labor knew that the dose of morphine was too small to stop the pain. Patients felt it, but because of the scopolamine they did not remember it. Some observers reported hearing parturients scream from several floors or several houses away. To physicians accustomed to dealing with patients quietly anesthetized with ether or chloroform, Twilight Sleep must have seemed a poor substitute. Nor did scopolamine reliably provide the degree of amnesia that Gauss had claimed. As many as one in five of Gauss's own patients had memories of pain even when he used his special memory test to adjust doses. Williams, DeLee, and others had good reason to complain that the method was too inconsistent to be useful.

And there were other problems. The first preparations of scopolamine were chemically unstable and required special handling. Patients treated with it required an extra person to watch them, but hospitals often did not have enough nurses or physicians to provide the individual care that the women needed and that increased the cost of childbirth. Although the wealthy might be able to afford Twilight Sleep, poorer women could not, and it was, in any case, hardly the boon that the founders of the National Twilight Sleep Association had hoped it might be.

The National Twilight Sleep Association

For almost a full year after publication of Tracy and Leupp's original article in *McClure's,* the campaign for Twilight Sleep increased in intensity. Then, almost as suddenly, the movement collapsed. Several events contributed to its demise. A major one was the death of Mrs. Carmody.[28]

Mrs. Carmody had been one of the strongest, most active, and most visible supporters of Twilight Sleep, often displaying her own Freiburg Baby at department store rallies. She and her lawyer husband had even founded a special Twilight Sleep hospital in Brooklyn. When Mrs. Carmody died during her second labor, her physician and her husband attributed the death to hemorrhage and not to a complication of Twilight Sleep. These assurances notwithstanding, the public remained concerned, particularly because hemorrhage was one of the complications that had most worried obstetricians cautious about Twilight Sleep. The *New York Times* reported Mrs. Carmody's death and published her husband's statement and the comment of Alice J. Olson of Flatbush, who lamented that she had wanted to warn her friend of the danger of Twilight Sleep but had failed to do so. Alice Olson publicly vowed to campaign against Twilight Sleep. Following this news report, the next, and last, editorial on the subject in the *Times* mentioned many of the medical objections to Twilight Sleep and suggested that the issue should be resolved on the basis of fact rather than opinion.[29]

World War I was another event that decreased the popularity of Twilight Sleep. The campaign for Twilight Sleep had begun in 1914 just as German and Allied forces sent their first troops into the trenches of Belgium and France. Animosity toward "the Hun" escalated as newspapers carried stories of new atrocities. Interest in Twilight Sleep simultaneously waned, although there were sporadic reports of American women who found their way through enemy lines so that they could deliver under Gauss's care.

Most of all, Twilight Sleep failed because it did not fulfill public expectations. Claims for its effectiveness had been overblown, only to succumb to the persistent skepticism of most physicians. As one New York obstetrician observed, "Every new method of treatment is subject to all the dangers to which a first and only child is exposed. It is spoiled by too much praise and killed with kindness." American patients learned what Europeans had known a decade earlier: there is no panacea for the pain of labor. In an article published in 1929, even Gauss took a more moderate position.[30]

The national campaign for Twilight Sleep died, but the method did not disappear. Various modifications were used for almost another half-century. As physicians became more accustomed to it, they became more bold with doses. Within a decade they had forgotten the admonitions of Gauss, Williams, and DeLee; they gave larger and larger amounts of opioids and even combined Twilight Sleep with general and spinal anesthesia. Medical papers no longer ascribed arrested labor, neonatal depression, or maternal hemorrhage to use of these drugs. Ironically, the event that brought a decisive end to the clinical use of Twilight Sleep was another public campaign, one that began in 1960 out of concern for the potentially harmful effects of drugs on the infant.

In retrospect, the confrontation between the American public and physicians in 1914 had little chance for resolution. American women were motivated by a social philosophy that placed a high value on personal comfort and by an extraordinary faith that science could conquer pain. Physicians, on the other hand, ignored the social issues and dealt with the problem as one to be resolved by experimentation and the collection of clinical data. Physicians never addressed the social issues, and patients discounted many of the medical problems.

"Labor Is Pathogenic"

The National Birthday Trust Fund Campaign
in Great Britain

It is no use people saying our grandmothers had babies

without anaesthetics. Women's standards are different today.

The modern woman is not going to accept the standards

of the nineteenth century. Science has proved that it

can make things easier for them and they want

the help that science can give them.

—*Daily Mirror,* May 1945

In 1927, thirteen years after the formation of the National Twilight Sleep Association in the United States, a similar campaign began in Great Britain. On the surface, the two were very similar in motivation and goals, but the impact on medical practice was very different, primarily because the British public activists used very different methods to achieve their objectives.

As with its American predecessor, the National Birthday Trust Fund was founded and directed by upper-class women. "Incensed by the injustice" of a system that gave only wealthy women access to good care, Lady Cholmondeley and Lady Rhys-Williams started the organization "with the object of raising funds for the extension of Maternity Services and of undertaking inquiries and investigations under medical supervision, which might point the way to the permanent solution of the problems of safe and painless Motherhood." The organization focused on three issues: increasing the availability of health services for poor women, improving nutrition for young children, and relieving the pain of childbirth. Within a year Lucy, Countess Baldwin of Bewdeley, wife of Prime Minister Stanley Baldwin, assumed responsibility for the fund's efforts to improve the availability of obstetric anesthesia. She later formed the Anaesthetic Appeal Fund, an organization separate from, but affiliated with, the National Birthday Trust Fund. Through the work of Lady Baldwin and Lady Rhys-Williams, the campaign for obstetric anesthesia became the liveliest and most visible activity of the fund. The anesthesia division organized benefits to raise money from the aristocracy and used radio talks, lectures, and pamphlets to elicit support from the general population.[1]

The fund, in its repudiation of pain, its faith in medical technology, and its tone of moral rectitude, resembled many social movements of the previous century. One pamphlet contained the question "Is it natural and right that a mother should endure pain when a baby is born?" The answer was, of course, no, and anyone who opposed anesthesia was chided, regardless of the reason for opposing it. "There are still a few people who believe that pain is a natural adjunct of childbirth and that artificial means of relieving it are wrong. Another school of thought holds that childbirth can and should be painless if regarded by the mother as a natural and normal process. Most people, including the majority of doctors, agree that childbearing is naturally a process incurring varying degrees of pain differing in intensity from one patient to another. It is agreed that it is wrong and unnecessary that any mother should be allowed to suffer when there are methods available to relieve pain without causing harm to herself and the baby."[2]

As in the United States, the campaign in Great Britain for ameliorating the dangers of childbirth emerged from the feminist movement. Thus, John Stuart Mill, who had written a harsh description of labor pain, became an early and ardent advocate of woman's rights.[3] In an era when many women bore six or more children, feminists believed that liberation from the mental, physical, and social burdens of childbearing and childrearing was at least as important as political and economic enfranchisement. Education offered some hope for control over family size, and anesthesia promised freedom from debilitating fear and pain. Hospitalization for childbirth meant respite from family responsibilities for the duration of convalescence. Good maternal care would, moreover, probably enhance a woman's life for years to come. Delivery by a skillful practitioner meant less risk of developing a recto-vaginal fistula, for instance, or a prolapsed bladder.

Leaders of the National Birthday Trust Fund identified the welfare of all women as a goal of their organization. Absent was the nineteenth- century assumption that women who had less education or social refinement experienced less physical pain and, therefore, needed less help. All women suffer, they thought, but only the privileged few had the financial resources to cope. One English author, Vera Brittain, reflecting on her experience with childbirth in 1927, wrote: "This is what nine-tenths of the mothers in this country go through—not once, but again and again. Even now, I don't really know what they suffer. It was just a mistake that I was given no alleviation for the pain, and could come back to a pleasant home with people to help me. But they have to be up in a few days, and do everything for the baby and everyone else."[4] Like the American socialites who established the National Twilight Sleep Association, the founders of the National Birthday Trust Fund had an egalitarian compassion for all women.

Joseph DeLee and Obstetric Care

The medical goals of English feminists fit well with trends in obstetrics. Since the turn of the century, obstetricians in Great Britain, as in the United States, had emphasized prenatal maternal care as a form of preventive medicine. A prominent leader of this movement was Joseph B. DeLee, an American obstetrician who had opposed Twilight Sleep. Born to impoverished immigrant parents, DeLee devoted his career to improving the care of Chicago's poor. He developed programs to teach obstetrics to medical students and to provide obstetric care to immigrant women. He also founded the Chicago Lying-In Hospital and Dispensary.[5] DeLee was a strong advocate of the active management of childbirth, and his ideas influenced physicians throughout the Western world. Among other things, he recommended ether anesthesia for delivery because this allowed him to perform procedures that otherwise would have been impossible because of the pain, such as an episiotomy, stimulation of the uterus with oxytocin or ergots, use of forceps for delivery of the child, manual extraction of the placenta from the uterine cavity, and surgical repair of the episiotomy.

DeLee's philosophy signaled a radical departure from the watchful expectancy that had characterized obstetric practice in the previous century. Nineteenth-century physicians had called childbirth a natural process, one that rarely justified medical intervention. Meigs had criticized Simpson on just these grounds, calling anesthesia for a normal delivery unnecessarily intrusive.

DeLee acknowledged that his method "interferes much with Nature's process." Citing the frequency of serious complications with normal deliveries, however, he doubted the benefits of restraint. "A dismal outcome" was so common, he said, that he

> often wondered whether Nature did not deliberately intend women should be used up in the process of reproduction, in a manner analogous to that of the salmon, which dies after spawning. Perhaps laceration, prolapse and all the evils are, in fact, natural to labor and therefore normal, in the same way as the death of the mother salmon and the death of the male bee in copulation, are natural and normal. If you adopt this view, I have no ground to stand on, but, if you believe that a woman after delivery should be as healthy, as well and anatomically perfect as she was before, and that the child should

be undamaged, then you will have to agree with me that labor is pathogenic, because experience has proved such ideal results exceedingly rare.[6]

Other obstetricians agreed with DeLee. Austin Flint asked how a "process that kills thousands of women each year, leaves a quarter of all cases more or less invalided, is attended by severe pain and tearing of tissues, and kills three to seven percent of all babies, can be called a normal or physiologic function?" Another was George Engelmann, the obstetrician whose descriptions of birthing practices of "savages" two decades earlier had justified greater use of anesthesia for "civilized" women.[7]

Many obstetricians in both Great Britain and the United States thought that aggressive management would decrease the incidence of complications. Speaking to colleagues, one obstetrician promised: "You and I, in making the effort to make it [labor] painless, are going to spend more time with our patients. We are going to watch the fetal heart very carefully. We are going to detect the signs of impending danger. As a result, we are going to have a lowered infant mortality, and the tremendous morbidity will gradually be eliminated." Following this philosophy, obstetricians performed more operative procedures. At one prominent New York hospital, forceps deliveries increased fourfold between 1890 and 1950.[8] The use of anesthesia and the need for hospital beds also increased.

Obstetricians and feminists found, therefore, that their goals coincided, but they also found that other segments of society did not share their vision, including other physicians.

Obstacles to the Use of Obstetric Anesthesia

Of the obstacles to obstetric anesthesia leaders of the National Birthday Trust Fund identified government policies as the most troublesome. Even before 1948, the year that Great Britain nationalized medical care, activists held the government responsible for health care. Brittain railed about it in her book *Testament of Experience*, written in the aftermath of World War I. "Government after government insists that we can't afford a national maternity service—we who spend millions a year on armaments to destroy the bodies which are produced at such cost. At such time I was filled with a vehement anger. I wanted to batter down the solid walls of the Ministry of Health; to take the Minister himself and give him a woman's insides, and compel him to have six babies, all without anaesthetics." In a similar vein, Virginia Woolf suggested that one advantage of the political empowerment of women would be a government that provides "every mother with chloroform when the child is born." It is noteworthy that both the National Twilight Sleep Association and the National Birthday Trust Fund were each formed just a few years before women in America and England, respectively, won the right to vote (1919 and 1931).[9]

Public ambivalence was another obstacle. Some women were indifferent to the use of anesthesia, and others still believed it sinful to relieve the pain of childbirth by artificial means. Many women feared anesthesia because they associated it with obstetric emergencies.[10]

Medical tradition was a third obstacle. Existing law forbade midwives to administer drugs other than a handful of sedatives, drugs that cause drowsiness without relieving pain. This was of little practical use. Physicians could give anesthetics, but few attended a delivery unless a special problem arose. Among family practitioners, the group most likely to be called, many thought anesthesia undesirable for labor. Conservative by inclination and training, they perpetuated many of the attitudes toward sex and gender that feminists hoped to change. The historian Susan Kent suggests that the stodginess of physicians often made them the special target of feminists.[11]

The Campaign of the National Birthday Trust Fund

The campaign organized by the National Birthday Trust Fund was sophisticated and comprehensive. It relied heavily on the news media to publicize the work of the fund and to expose the deficiencies of the government. Early in the campaign, newspapers showed pictures of social functions that the fund sponsored to raise money from the aristocracy. Later, articles described the poor anesthesia services provided by local medical councils and praised the efforts of the fund to counteract that deficiency. An article in the *Daily Express* reported that "the ordinary woman of this country still has to have her baby without relief. She cannot afford a nursing home and there is little room in the hospitals. The midwife who attends her either is not qualified to administer an anaesthetic or has not the apparatus. In 1940 only 44 of 188 local councils provided even one machine. The doctor often is too indifferent or too busy. It is left to a private charity organization to do the pioneer work." An article in the *Daily Mirror* described how "red tape and the die hard attitudes of local authorities are responsible for the pain and suffering each day in child-birth of hundreds of British mothers."[12]

Newspapers increased public interest by reporting social inequities in the existing medical system. One story, "Mothers Want the Princess' Drugs," told how "every expectant mother should soon benefit by the two pain-killing drugs which were available for Princess Elizabeth [later queen, giving birth, in 1948, to her first son, Charles]. They are pethidine [an opioid], for the early stages of labor, and trilene [an anesthetic gas], administered before the birth. The National Birthday Trust Fund is urging that every midwife in the country should be allowed to use both drugs when attending cases on her own." Alluding both to social inequities and to government indifference, Virginia Woolf wrote: "Since chloroform was first administered to Queen Victoria on the birth of Prince Leopold in April 1853, normal maternity cases in the wards have had to wait for seventy-six years and the advocacy of the Prime Minister's wife to obtain this relief." [13]

Newspapers generated even more support when they admonished women to unite against government officials. "If you think all this is wrong, it is up to you to do something about it! Get at your maternity and child welfare doctor (he is your contact with the Ministry of Health) and tell him what you think," one article read. Another writer said: "Women's organizations throughout the country should make themselves heard upon this matter now. It is essential that the new National Health Services scheme should include the provision of adequate relief for every mother. They will not do unless mothers demand it. They [women] should organize themselves at once to demand this simple and vital reform. It is a slur on our humanity that we allow our mothers to suffer quite unnecessarily out of sheer inertia and slackness in providing available relief." [14]

As the publicity campaign continued, the National Birthday Trust Fund developed extensive support among sympathetic professionals. At one time, the organization could boast a general committee "comprised of eminent medical men and women, specialists in obstetrics, gynaecologists and anaesthetists, pioneer social welfare workers, representatives of women's organizations, and nursing and midwifery associations, and of lay people to whom the welfare of mothers is of great concern."[15] No doubt the political and social connections of the founders of the fund helped them to recruit volunteers.

The fund developed a particularly important alliance with the College of Obstetricians and Gynaecologists. For the college, the association was established at a most propitious time. A pall had engulfed obstetrics since the eighteenth century, when physicians had first sought a greater role in the delivery of babies. Medical schools taught obstetrics poorly. A physician rarely attended a delivery unless the patient was wealthy or a midwife required special assistance. Often the physician who responded was less experienced than the midwife who had summoned him. In spite of improvements in other areas of medicine, maternal death rates in England had barely changed since the nineteenth century. Reminiscing, the Scottish obstetrician Sir Dugald Baird remarked: "In the Glasgow Royal Maternity Hospital in the 1920s, there was an average of two maternal deaths every week, and we were so preoccupied with the problem of keeping the mother alive that the very high foetal mortality was very seldom discussed." Several European countries had improved obstetric training sooner and had better statistics than Great Britain, and the public knew of these disparities. For good reason, then, neither other medical professionals nor the laity in Great Britain held obstetrics in high regard.[16]

Sensing widespread public displeasure, Parliament initiated reforms. In 1902 it enacted the first of several regulations designed to improve training and raise standards for the certification of midwives. At the same time, obstetricians worked to enhance instruction in and practice of their specialty.[17] Overcoming significant political opposition from the Royal Colleges of Physicians and Surgeons, resistant to the perceived undermining of their authority, obstetricians formed the College of Obstetricians and Gynaecologists in 1929. Within another nine years and after considerably more political preparation and work, the organization was finally designated a *Royal* College, a formality that enhanced the status of the specialty.

Founded around the same time, the National Birthday Trust Fund and the College of Obstetricians and Gynaecologists both needed to establish themselves with the public. The fund wanted better care for mothers, and obstetricians thought that they were the group best able to provide that care. The fund needed allies for its battle against government bureaucracy, and the college needed public recognition from a highly respected private organization. Both the fund and the college needed to convince rank-and-file practitioners, the group of physicians whom they thought should be delivering most babies, of the benefits of better obstetric care and the advantages of anesthesia.[18] The strengths and needs of the two organizations therefore dovetailed nicely.

To improve obstetric anesthesia, the fund undertook several medical projects. One supported Louis Carnac Rivett, a consulting obstetrician at Queen Charlotte's Hospital. Rivett helped develop a small glass capsule that could be broken to release a measured amount of chloroform onto a face mask. The chloroform relieved some of the pain of labor—that is, it provided analgesia—without causing unconsciousness. The fund paid for the manufacture of capsules and helped to distribute them free or at cost to hospitals serving poor communities. The fund even sent capsules to Commonwealth countries that could not obtain them otherwise.[19]

Another project helped R. J. Minnitt, an anesthesiologist who had developed an apparatus that could deliver a fixed, safe dose of nitrous oxide. The medical effects of nitrous oxide had been known since the early nineteenth century, and as early as 1880 a Russian physician, Stanislav C. Kliklowicz, had suggested its use for labor pain.[20] Several characteristics of nitrous oxide made it ideal for obstetrics. It was odorfree and pleasant to breathe. Low concentrations of nitrous oxide relieved pain even while patients remained awake, so patients benefited from the analgesic properties of the drug without being anesthetized. Analgesia started almost with the patient's first breath and ended just as quickly after they stopped breathing the agent. Unfortunately, nitrous oxide was difficult to administer, and for years that problem kept obstetricians from using nitrous oxide for their patients.

Minnitt circumvented technical difficulties by modifying an apparatus to administer anesthesia that had been developed several years earlier by an American anesthesiologist. Minnitt designed a valve that delivered a predetermined mixture of nitrous oxide and air whenever the patient placed a mask to her face and pressed a lever. Should inhalation of nitrous oxide make the patient too sleepy, she would be unable to hold the mask or depress the lever and would awaken. Minnitt's apparatus allowed each woman to decide when she needed pain relief and how much. This eliminated the need for a trained anesthesiologist, an important consideration because few were available in Great Britain. Minnitt's first anesthetic machines, which were large and cumbersome, could only be used in hospitals, a significant restriction because more than 80 percent of British women still delivered their babies at home or in small maternity units. With support from the fund, John Elam, another anesthesiologist, made Minnitt's apparatus smaller and lighter so that it could be carried into homes. As with the capsules of chloroform, the fund bought these gas-air machines and helped distribute them to poor communities.[21]

In other projects, the National Birthday Trust Fund sought drugs to replace ether, chloroform, and morphine, all of which had significant disadvantages for labor. By 1950 the fund had sponsored clinical trials of paraldehyde, an early sedative; trichlorethylene, an inhalation agent; and meperidine (called pethidine in Great Britain) and alphaprodine, two synthetic opioids. At the suggestion of officers of the Royal College of Obstetricians and Gynaecologists, the fund also sponsored research to evaluate the safety of various anesthetic methods for the pain of childbirth.[22]

The fund helped increase the number of people able to administer obstetric anesthesia. By donating money to employ six anesthesiologists for maternity units, it improved care in select London hospitals, but this had little effect on the overall problem. The fund sought another solution as well. It lobbied Parliament to change laws governing midwives so that they might administer opium and use Rivett's chloroform capsules and Minnitt's gas-air apparatus, and it worked with the Central Midwives' Board to create programs to train midwives to administer analgesic concentrations of gas, to develop criteria to assess their competence, and to design studies to evaluate the efficacy of the program. Seeking even wider influence for its work, the fund sponsored visits by nurses from other countries to English obstetric units.[23]

The fund's projects relieved some medical problems but uncovered others. Some of the new drugs did not provide adequate analgesia, so during prolonged labor a woman could receive dangerous amounts of chloroform from repeated use of the capsules. In one instance, a physician entered a labor room to find that his patient had crushed the glass capsule between her teeth and had swallowed the chloroform. Minnitt's original apparatus caused maternal and fetal hypoxia. When Minnitt designed the machine, obstetricians were not concerned about oxygenation of the fetus and did not consider the potential danger of having the mother breathe air diluted by a high concentration of nitrous oxide. When later models of the apparatus substituted oxygen for air, the addition of a heavy tank of compressed oxygen reduced the portability of the machine. Portability had always been a problem. Even the small machines developed by Elam weighed fifty pounds. Midwives could not balance the devices on their bicycle carriers, and local medical councils were reluctant to pay a taxicab to transport the machines, particularly because midwives were expected to ride their own bicycles to the homes of patients in labor.[24]

Changes in Medical Practice

Judged by virtually any criteria, the National Birthday Trust Fund was a success. Early victories were small: local councils endorsed the idea of better services and more anesthesia. In 1934, for example, the Maternity and Child Welfare Committee of the Hertfordshire County called maternal suffering "a national problem" and said that it believed "strongly that in all maternity cases the use of gas and air analgesia should be available as far as it lies in the power of the committee so to arrange." The committee feared that the Royal Commission might take another twenty years to reform this situation but suggested that "ordinary women could get the reform started now."[25] From such modest starts, public enthusiasm increased. Within two decades the central government was fully committed to improvements in women's health care.

How much did obstetric anesthesia change in the 1930s and 1940s in Great Britain? In 1929 a senior public health official, Dr. Laetitia Fairfield, reported that London maternity units had delivered 7,454 women the preceding year. No more than one in twenty of these mothers had received a sedative or analgesic for normal labor, and even fewer had received a general anesthetic, and only then in the event of some major obstetric problem. In fact, only eleven of twenty-two London obstetric units surveyed had offered any form of relief for normal delivery—even though obstetric care in London was reputed to be the best available in the country, a fact that illustrates the situation elsewhere. By 1948, in contrast, 288 of 295 obstetric units throughout the country offered some form of anesthesia for normal deliveries. Moreover, 50 percent of women who delivered in hospitals and 8 percent of women who delivered at home received some form of anesthesia. A member of Parliament, Edith Somerskill, said, "Enlightened hospitals do give anaesthetics."[26]

There were improvements, then, in the overall availability of anesthesia, but social and geographic inequities remained. A report of a special committee of the Royal College of Obstetricians and Gynaecologists noted that wives of professional people received anesthesia for delivery twice as often as wives of manual laborers; and women living in England or Scotland received anesthesia twice as often as women living in Wales.[27]

The report also noted that English women wanted better service. In 1945, in fifteen thousand interviews conducted shortly after delivery, women complained most often about their difficulties in obtaining adequate relief of labor pain. Clearly, public apathy and fear of anesthesia had diminished.

Similar resistance from the medical community had also

diminished, as suggested by the fact that physicians' wives were one group that received anesthesia for their deliveries. Women physicians themselves used anesthesia for their own labors: during a five-year period 221 reported receiving anesthesia for more than half of their 410 deliveries. Comments about obstetric anesthesia at medical meetings also became more enthusiastic. As one physician said, "It behooves us as physicians to put forth our strongest efforts to make labor less of a burden for the average woman. We should make it as painless as we can."[28]

Grudgingly, physicians and local medical councils expanded their support programs to train midwives to administer anesthesia.[29] Within five years, the program developed jointly by the Central Midwives Bureau and the National Birthday Trust Fund had trained 27,583 midwives. Within another ten years, that number had almost doubled. Within two decades of the founding of the National Birthday Trust Fund, public support and demand for obstetric anesthesia had increased dramatically.

A Comparison of Campaigns

The National Birthday Trust Fund and the National Twilight Sleep Association not only began about the same time but were both outgrowths of the nineteenth-century feminist movement and were both founded by upper-class women who believed better health to be an important part of emancipation. Both organizations succeeded in increasing public awareness of obstetric anesthesia, and both influenced medical practice. By 1950 support for obstetric anesthesia was greater in Great Britain and the United States than it had ever been in the past.

But there were also differences between the organizations. The accomplishments of the National Birthday Trust Fund seem more substantial in scope. In the course of its work, it influenced government policy, educated the public, and involved physicians in its campaign. It sponsored surveys, improved medical technology, funded positions for anesthesiologists at maternity units and hospitals, and even served as a charitable organization, dispensing money, equipment, and drugs to needy communities. It sustained these activities for several decades.

A number of factors contributed to the fund's success. First, unlike the National Twilight Sleep Association, which sought only to establish Twilight Sleep, the fund worked to improve all aspects of women's health care. The campaign for obstetric anesthesia, its most visible activity, was just one part of an overall campaign. Second, the fund worked well with other groups. Whereas the National Twilight Sleep Association had attacked physicians, the fund developed strong relationships with groups that could help—government officials, obstetricians, and anesthesiologists—even recruiting them to participate in the solution of the problems. Third, the fund never became enmeshed in the resolution of technical issues. It encouraged physicians to decide which methods of anesthesia were safest and most appropriate. In fact, because of research from one medical study the fund even withdrew its support for chloroform capsules. In contrast, American activists promoted Twilight Sleep despite the objections of physicians.

In fairness to the American women who formed the National Twilight Sleep Association, let me point out that this situation was different. For example, physicians had new ways to relieve the pain. One paper written in 1933 listed eleven different drugs or techniques, and this did not include local anesthesia or such regional techniques as spinal anesthesia and sacral and presacral blocks, which many obstetricians had tried. Caudal anesthesia, a variant of regional anesthesia, was popularized by an American anesthesiologist, Robert Hingson. These new techniques of regional anesthesia were backed by recent, extensive studies of the anatomy and physiology of pelvic nerves.[30]

No less important, physicians thought differently about obstetric anesthesia, and for this the National Twilight Sleep Association can take some of the credit. Physicians, like every other group, respond to social pressure. Patients influence practice by employing physicians who provide services that the patients want. An emotional statement by one American obstetrician describes the new climate.

> Every expectant mother has the right to demand the safe and painless conduct of labor which modern obstetrics makes possible. As long as ignorance regarding the facts in the case remains so general among the mothers of this country; as long as Christian Scientists and those who complacently point out that their grandmothers and the Indians and the mothers of Central Africa got along without prenatal care and without modern obstetricians, keep the mothers of our own country from seeking the protection of these modern blessings and from securing by united efforts the passage of necessary laws which would make it incumbent on the communities, the states, or the national Government to make proper provisions for all expectant mothers, rich and poor, alike; just how long will the untold suffering, the waste of thousands of infants' lives, the immeasurable damage to health and mind, fill our hospitals and our institutions for the blind and feeble-minded and continue to go unchecked.[31]

The resounding success of feminist activists during the first half of the twentieth century tends to obscure the beginning of the next movement in obstetric care. Sown in the success of their campaign for anesthesia were the seeds that would lead to its dissolution. In spite of changing patterns of medical practice, large segments of the public and the medical profession harbored doubts about the benefits of, and the need for, obstetric anesthesia.

DeLee's advocacy of aggressive obstetric practices precipitated a storm of criticism. For example, J. Whitridge Williams decried this approach, citing problems of infection, hemorrhage, and dysfunctional labor, many of which he attributed to overuse of anesthesia. Other obstetricians who felt just as strongly suggested that every unnecessary intrusion into the normal process of labor evoked a whole new set of problems, which then had to be addressed by even more aggressive management. One wrote: "It was a natural consequence that all obstetric procedures had their indications widened as their relative safety became established. But that any operation, because asepsis makes it reasonably safe and anesthesia keeps the patient quiet during its performance, should be so inordinately broadened in its scope that the suspicion is evidence that it is being done for the convenience and conservation of time of the operator, is a travesty on scientific endeavor." In this same vein, the English obstetrician James Young once observed: "There can be no doubt that the present well-intentioned attempts to bring the advantages of anesthesia in greater measure to the woman in labor frequently tend to fix the doctor still more firmly to the obstetric machine under conditions which are neither satisfactory to himself nor in the best interests of his patient. The increasing recourse to hospital for delivery, which is so common a feature of many modern communities, constitutes another major obstetric problem." In effect, DeLee's ideas about active management reopened the nineteenth-century obstetric controversy about meddlesome practices. Once again obstetricians argued the nature of normal labor, the role of the obstetrician, and the significance of labor pain. In effect, the relative dangers and benefits of anesthesia lay at the heart of the dispute, just as they had in Simpson's day.[32]

Some segments of the public also disliked the trend toward hospital deliveries and anesthetized labor. In the 1948 report *Maternity in Great Britain,* several women mentioned that they preferred to deliver at home rather than in a hospital because they "felt safer," because they "wanted to stay with my child and husband and be able to see my friends," or because they wanted some close relative with them during the delivery. Six percent of women interviewed refused anesthesia because they did not need relief, because they did not wish to "blow into that mask thing," or because they were afraid.[33]

Professional and public dissatisfaction eventually coalesced into the movement advocating "natural childbirth." Formally, this movement may date from 1933, just four years after Lady Cholmondeley and Lady Rhys-Williams began the National Birthday Trust Fund. The instigator of the new movement was Grantly Dick Read, a colorful, charismatic, and persuasive English obstetrician. Although using medical facts in controversial ways, Read's message found great favor among a new generation of patients. To many physicians, however, Read raised fears that science would disappear from obstetric practice.

CHAPTER TEN

"As God Intended"

Grantly Dick Read and the Natural Childbirth Movement

To me this work is no longer an obstetric practice only, but a

mission—no longer a pursuit, but a calling. I am not a holy

person, but sincerely believe that time has shown clearly that

the only justification for my professional existence is to give

everything to spread the Gospel of sane and happy childbirth.

—Grantly Dick Read, unpublished manuscript, circa 1948

The natural childbirth movement in England was a trend away from the use of forceps, ergots, and anesthesia, which had begun almost a century earlier. The man responsible for the shift was Grantly Dick Read, an English obstetrician practicing in Woking, just outside London. Read combined old principles of obstetrics with a smattering of science, which he served to the public with a generous sprinkling of Victorian romanticism. Read's method appealed to women who were dissatisfied with the regimentation of modern obstetric care and to those obstetricians who had never believed in the benefits of the aggressive management of childbirth. Read repelled other physicians, however, who thought his ideas simplistic, if not incorrect, and his style flamboyant.

Stimulated by opposition and buoyed by a mystical faith in motherhood, Read made his career a quest to change obstetric practice. In one sense he succeeded. "Natural childbirth," as he called his method, became a household phrase. His most important book, *Childbirth Without Fear,* was published in several languages, and educational programs patterned after his methods appeared around the world.[1] By the time of his death in 1959, Read had altered many obstetric practices, including the management of pain. Yet despite public acclaim, Read never received the professional recognition that he thought he deserved—probably because he had created a schism between women patients and their physicians.

Read's Vision of Natural Childbirth

According to Grantly Dick Read, "Healthy childbirth was never intended by the natural law to be painful." Normally,

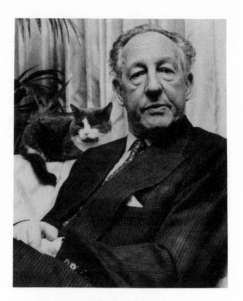

Grantly Dick Read (1890–1959).
Courtesy of the Wellcome Institute
Library, London.

birth is "carried out by natural processes from beginning to end, influenced by natural emotions and perfected by the harmony of the mechanism [with the woman] conscious throughout the progress of her baby's birth, so that she can truly fulfill herself emotionally when she sees and welcomes the child emerging from her womb into the world." To Read, natural childbirth also meant that the "baby is not separated from its mother and placed in a communal nursery [and] that she can have her husband with her during her baby's birth."[2]

Read believed that the art of natural childbirth had been lost, except among "women of the more primitive types." He attributed the success of such women to the superior conditioning of their bodies by a life of hard physical work and to

their innate understanding of the biological and social significance of childbirth.

> [Primitive women are] rarely troubled by anxiety states
> or toxic manifestations. Malaise or sickness seldom pre-
> vents them from continuing such work as they are in the
> habit of performing. The primitive knows that she will
> have little trouble when her child is born. She knows that
> it will be small and healthy, and she has no knowledge
> of bones misshapen by rickets disease and faulty habits
> during childhood. Natural birth is all that she looks for;
> there are no fears in her mind; no midwives spoiling the
> natural process; she has no knowledge of the tragedies
> of sepsis, infection and hemorrhage. To have conceived
> is her joy; the ultimate result of her conception is her
> ambition. Eventually, and probably whilst even yet at her
> work, labor commences. . . . There is unquestionably a
> sense of satisfaction when she feels the first symptoms
> and receives the impatiently awaited indications that her
> child is about to arrive . . . [she] isolates herself, and, in
> a thicket, quietly and undisturbed she patiently waits.

Those who die, "two, three or four percent of some tribes
[do so] without any sadness, realizing if they were not competent to produce children for the spirits of their fathers and
for the tribe, they had no place in the tribe."[3]

Read believed that "primitives" have no inherent physical advantage over "moderns," and attributed the success of
primitive women to their state of mind. Modern women,
Read said, had lost their competence for natural childbirth
through the cumulative effects of acculturation. "From the
earliest childhood, the modern cultured girl is brought up
protected from the hard facts of life. . . . She is rarely called

upon to use her natural instincts . . . alas, reproduction does not move with civilization, and parturition is almost invariably the first primitive, fundamental physical act which she is called upon to perform."[4]

Among the factors that distort a woman's natural instincts regarding childbirth, Read included the Victorian proclivity for secrecy about sex, the dissemination of false information by friends and relatives, the exaggeration of childbirth pain that appeared in books such as Vera Brittain's *Honourable Estate* (1936), and the religious teachings that labor pain is just punishment for sin. Read believed that fear increased obstetric problems and that pain itself could cause permanent physical damage to the woman. Read also said that modern obstetric practices disrupted childbirth and increased its risks. "It is generally agreed that one of the most important factors in the production of complicated labor and, therefore, of maternal and infantile mortality, is the inability of obstetricians and midwives to stand by and allow the natural and uninterrupted course of labor. . . . It is an unquestionable fact that interference is still one of the greatest dangers with which both the mother and child have to contend." A natural childbirth, as advocated by Read, consisted of eliminating unnecessary medical interference. He told obstetricians and midwives to deliver women "as God intended"—that is, without anesthesia, forceps, or other meddlesome medical practices. He told women to prepare their bodies with exercise and to prepare their minds with information and mental techniques.[5]

Read publicized his ideas through books, pamphlets, lectures, and a voluminous correspondence with patients, other physicians, and newspaper editors. Read wrote the first version of his book in 1919 but refrained from publication at his professor's suggestion that he first finish his obstetric training. The published version, *Natural Childbirth*, appeared in England in 1933 and its sequel, *Revelation of Childbirth*, in 1943. The latter book appeared in America two years later as *Childbirth Without Fear*, the title used for subsequent editions in both countries.[6]

Read's Vision of Motherhood

Motivating Read was a messianic vision of motherhood. Jessie, a former patient whom Read married after his divorce in 1952, described her husband as a "dedicated man" to whom "childbirth was a holy event—a spiritual and physical manifestation of all that is creatively beautiful within woman."[7] Read's unshakable conviction in the beauty of natural childbirth and in the "mother love" that springs from it was the inspiration for his quest.

Mother love, Read said, is a primal force, capable of permanently changing lives and shaping history. "No woman who remembers her child's birth ever ceases to love that child, and no child who has been born in love and learned of its mother's love, ever ceases to love its mother . . . and so more unselfish love will fill the world . . . and all the actions and ambitions of men and women will be influenced from selfishness to the path which is followed by love." Transformed by mother love, men and women would abolish "poverty, distress and misery among the masses" and would change the character of nations and, eventually, the world. All this must grow from the seed of mother love, an inevitable product, he believed, of a natural birth. Conversely, "the pain of labor and its initiating cause, fear, extend their evil influence into the very roots of our social structure. They corrupt the minds and bodies of successive generations and bring distress and calamity where happiness and prosperity are the natural reward of a simple physiological performance."[8] Thus, the goal of Read's obstetric mission was nothing less than a new world order. Although such idealism and sentimentality suggest a young man, Read was forty-nine years old when he wrote the above lines to his mother. His early plans to become a missionary may account for the intensity and fervor of his subsequent work.

Read's Message

Throughout his life, Read saved books, newspaper clippings, lecture notes, and letters pertaining to both professional and private activities. Much of the material is intensely personal; very little of it explains the origin of his ideas, and many of his stories seem more apocryphal than real. He writes, for example, that he first observed the deleterious effects of Victorian secrecy on childbirth while a boy on the family farm in Norfolk, England. Later, as an awestruck young medical officer during World War I, he recognized the potential for an easy and beautiful birth when he watched a Greek and then a Flemish woman "drop a quick one" in the fields, smile, and then resume work almost without interruption.[9]

The source of Read's ideas about "primitive" births is less clear. Although he learned something about tribal practices after moving to South Africa in 1948, he had formed his ideas long before, while living in England, where his entire obstetric experience consisted of one year of training at University College Hospital in London and ten years of private practice in nearby Woking. Neither situation offered many opportunities to deliver babies of "primitive women." Opportunities were probably equally scarce after he moved to South Africa, where he had an urban practice. Read lamented the speed with which tribal women adopted European customs. "I have seen them come into a maternity hospital, well on in labor, and demand 'the needle' . . . don't go to the towns to learn about Africans . . . they have already become the flotsam of the torrent of the white man's infiltration." Read's definition of "primitives" presents yet another problem. He does not define the word and includes in the category women from "Hindustan, China, India and Japan" despite the cultural sophistication of these cultures.[10]

Equally personal are Read's stories about the effect of the mind on the pain of childbirth. Exhausted by the trench warfare of World War I and almost in shell shock, Read learned from an Indian subaltern the protective value of mental relaxation techniques. *Progressive Relaxation,* a book by Edmund Jacobson, helped Read refine these ideas. Read credits J. N. Langley and H. K. Anderson, two highly respected English physiologists, with teaching him about the sympathetic nervous system. From Sir Charles Sherrington's book *The Integrative Action of the Nervous System,* Read learned about nociceptors. *The Wisdom of the Body,* by the Harvard physiologist W. B. Cannon, introduced him to the physiologic concept of "fight or flight." Finally, papers in the Read archives at Wellcome Institute dated 1944 to 1945 contain notes about forty-three scientific articles on pain. Several papers were already more than sixty years old when Read's book appeared in 1933, but others had not been written and could not have contributed to his original ideas. Considering the material available to Read in 1933, the list is sparse, and, in any case, Read found this scientific material confusing and contradictory. He preferred to rely more on common sense and clinical experience than on the experiments and opinions of experts.[11] His personal papers do, however, contain detailed notes on deliveries.

Although Read professed difficulty in interpreting scientific data, he often referred to physiologic concepts to support his ideas. Women who were frightened by labor activated a flight-or-fight response, he said, during which time they released such neurohumors as adrenaline. Neurohumors inhibited labor by causing the longitudinal muscles of the uterus to relax and the circular muscles to constrict. Spasm of the circular muscle prevented cervical dilation and descent of the child through the pelvis. If strong or prolonged, spasms could also cause ischemia, diminished blood flow to the uterine muscle, which in turn produced maternal pain and increased the risk of permanent hypoxic damage to the fetus. Eliminating this "fear-tension-pain syndrome," as he called it, would prevent this abnormal sequence: circular muscles would relax, longitudinal muscles could contract, the cervix would dilate quickly, without ischemia or pain, and the child would descend through the pelvis for delivery.[12]

It is strange that any physician resisted Read's theory, for it contained little that was new. Experts had long recognized the importance of a woman's mental state for a fast and safe delivery. As early as 1832 an English obstetrician, Thomas Denman, wrote:

> As the infirmities and particular state of the body have a powerful influence upon the mind, and as the affections of the mind have on various occasions a reciprocal effect upon the body, it might be reasonably expected that the progress of a labor should sometimes be forwarded or hindered by the passions. It is constantly found that the fear of a labor, or the same impression from any other cause at the time of labor, often lessens the energy of all the powers of the constitution and diminishes, or wholly suppresses for a time, the action of the parts concerned

in parturition. It is also observed that a cheerful flow of the spirits, which arises from the hope of a happy event, inspires women with an activity and a resolution which are extremely useful and favorable in that situation.

Denman described in detail the demeanor that attendants should adopt to create a supportive atmosphere. The American physician Samuel Bard had written similar comments in his textbook, published two decades before Denman's. Read knew of this philosophy and cited early authors who supported it.[13]

Obstetricians had also long argued the dangers of meddlesome obstetrics. This issue underlay debates about ergot toward the beginning of the nineteenth century and resurfaced when James Young Simpson introduced general anesthesia to obstetrics in 1847. Curiously, the arguments that Meigs used against anesthesia in 1847 are almost identical to those used by Read a century later. Meddling was the same charge levied against DeLee in 1920 by conservative obstetricians who objected to the routine use of such aggressive methods as episiotomy and manual exploration of the uterus even for normal deliveries.[14] When Read criticized meddlesome obstetrics, he thought that his position was a traditional stance in an ongoing debate. It puzzled, frustrated, and angered him that so many physicians found his suggestions controversial. Read never seemed to realize that his style may have irritated his colleagues more than his message.

Read's Style

An obituary in the *British Medical Journal* described Read as a "man of striking appearance and handsome presence

. . . a brilliant speaker, expounding his views with a single-minded enthusiasm which carried his audience with him . . . in private life . . . [he was] very gay and excellent company." Those less enthralled with Read mentioned his knack for self-aggrandizement. One critic observed in 1957 that Read rivaled James Dean, Liberace, and Elvis Presley in his ability to create mass hysteria and that he differed from those celebrities only because his work preceded theirs and probably would last much longer.[15]

On several occasions, Read's proclivity for publicity almost destroyed his career. Allegations of unprofessional advertising caused Read's partners in Woking to dissolve their group in 1938. Similar concerns ten years later may have prompted the newly formed National Health Service to deny him a hospital consultantship. Forced by this rebuff to move to South Africa, Read encountered a related problem there. Citing several irregularities, unprofessional promotion of his work among them, the South African Medical and Dental Registry tried to withhold licensure. Read contested the decision and won, but only after taking the matter to court.[16] Without his flair for publicity, Read's mission surely would have faltered.

Read had a talent for choosing whatever argument suited his purpose. The man who had once said that pagan religions were best, calling Christianity a major cause of childbirth fear and pain, also declared the New Testament "the greatest book upon health," saying, "If you read the Gospels or the teaching of St. Paul you will find an extraordinary thing, you will discover quite quickly that the New Testament is one of the soundest treatises you have ever read on physiology. You cannot find a modern theory of physiology which is not clearly known to have been recognized in the ethical application of Christianity." Read used physiologic principles to promote his work, but he also said that the emotional and psychological state of the mother during pregnancy had more influence on the subsequent development of the child than biochemistry or genetics. Read quoted scientific papers but, when convenient, disparaged them. In one lecture he ridiculed a colleague who had used electric stimulation to study components of labor pain. "Laugh with me, ladies and gentlemen," Read said. "We cannot obtain normal reactions by the production of abnormal states. . . . I know him quite well [and] I do not hesitate . . . in exhibiting a certain cynicism about his work." [17]

He often made conflicting statements. In 1943 he disparaged efforts of physicians to find better techniques, saying, "Walt Disney could hardly do justice to the Silly Symphony of Obstetric Analgesia." Yet in a 1946 paper he wrote, "I do not wish to disagree with the advocates of applied anaesthesia, whether it is caudal, inhalation or parenteral, for pain must be prevented or relieved. Every effort to make childbirth a painless function should be carefully considered." In the course of one paragraph in a 1959 edition of his book, Read praised Hingson's use of caudal anesthesia, then criticized it, describing how "thousands of normal labors have been mutilated by this dangerous and unjustifiable procedure" that robs women of an important spiritual experience. He concluded with an exhortation: "How long, oh, how long will this nonsense go on? Why do not at least some of these first class-brains settle down to try really harmless methods of preventing pain in labor? Can the scientific mind see no further than drugs and anesthetics?" Although Read maintained that he never said that "labor doesn't hurt," he did say that "for the perfect labor anaesthesia is unnecessary because there is no pain." He also said that his methods were successful more than 95 percent of the time, an estimate thought high even by some of Read's supporters.[18]

Read was contentious and often acted rashly. Leaders of the National Birthday Trust Fund wanted safer, happier deliveries for all women, but Read never acknowledged the value of their work. Instead, he criticized their methods, impugned their motives, and suggested that officers of the fund acted out of ignorance of the true nature of childbirth. "The administrators of the Birthday Trust should look into these matters if they are working seriously for pain relief in childbirth and not be guided by political motives of gynaecologists who rarely attend normal labour. . . . What sort of people rob women of the full joys of motherhood because of prejudice or worse? Is it not disgraceful to read that in a few areas, midwives are under some pressure to produce evidence that their mothers have received anaesthetics? Surely the safety of mothers and babies carries greater political capital than ministerial statistics of unwanted stupor?"[19]

Had Read been wiser, he might have worked with the fund rather than fought it. In spite of holding different views about the value of anesthesia, both he and members of the fund wished to improve the health and welfare of women. The fund had a record of flexibility, pragmatism, and the ability to work with a variety of people and organizations. If Read had convinced its leaders of the value of his methods, the fund probably would have supported him, too.

One key difference between Read and the fund was in their concepts of the ideal role of women. The fund held that women should ultimately be free to participate in all aspects of public life. Read, on the other hand, wanted women to stay at home caring for their children.

A good educational career should be provided for every woman, but behind all this social organization there should be recognition of domestic training to fit the girl to take her own place in the ranks of motherhood. . . . Woman fails when she ceases to desire the children for which she was primarily made. Her true emancipation lies in freedom to fulfill her biological purpose, to satisfy her physiological demand and sustain her philosophy, to the end that motherhood may be established as the supremely important factor in the organization and administration of our national and international relationships. It is along these lines only that the power of woman can be made indispensable in the affairs of state. . . . With adequate remuneration to maintain home and family and sufficient leisure to enjoy them, the majority of the demands on women would be met.[20]

It is ironic that natural childbirth, a process embraced by feminists later in the century, was initiated by a man who held very conventional ideas about the role of women as mothers and homemakers.

Reactions of Physicians

If many physicians opposed him, some did offer support. Joseph DeLee, the Chicago obstetrician who had opposed Twilight Sleep, approved of Read—a strange development in that DeLee's advocacy of aggressive obstetric techniques helped create more demand for obstetric anesthesia. Ignoring this inconsistency, Read dedicated a book to his colleague. In 1947 Read lectured at fourteen institutions in the United States. One of these was Johns Hopkins, where he had been invited to speak by Nicholson Eastman, chairman of obstetrics. Four years earlier, Eastman had written a letter to Read saying, "Your attitude toward childbearing is a most wholesome one and points to an ideal towards which we should strive. My former chief, the late Dr. J. Whitridge Williams, used to speak of your work with much interest." In 1946 Eastman had written a thoughtful and supportive critique of one of Read's few professional papers. Read received another invitation from Herbert Thoms, chairman of obstetrics at Yale. Subsequently, Thoms and several co-workers taught and used Read's methods and published several papers describing their work with those methods.[21] During this time, Helen Heardman, an English physiotherapist, began a program to teach relaxation techniques for childbirth and wrote a book describing her methods. Thoms and Heardman remained strong advocates of Read's methods, but Eastman did not.

Read failed with most physicians because when they pressed him for data he had none. His books cited experts known to the public: Sherrington, a Nobel Laureate; Langley and Anderson, well-known Cambridge physiologists; and Walter Cannon, a Harvard professor who had written a popular book on physiology. These references may have impressed patients, but they were not enough to satisfy physicians, who by 1940 were receiving considerable training in science in medical school. One physiologist wrote, "I find it so very difficult to get anything which one can by the remotest chance call Scientific Evidence from the other side. I go on hoping but even when it is apparently just within my grasp, it is whisked away." Similar comments appeared in professional journals. One physician wrote, "There is a tendency today to introduce all these [natural childbirth methods] as a national policy as if benefit therefrom were an established fact. Does childbearing require special training to be natural?" Another noted that Read's methods, far from being simple, were highly technical and difficult to teach. Yet another, a physician who was both an anesthesiologist and an avowed supporter of childbirth education, worried that the emphasis on natural childbirth would mean a return of public, professional, and government apathy toward the use of anesthesia for childbirth pain. Although she recommended childbirth education and taught a course in it herself, this physician thought that the benefits were primarily psychological and not physical.[22]

The most devastating criticism of Read appeared in a long article in the *Journal of the American Medical Association* in 1950. Two prominent American obstetricians challenged the statement that women of "less industrialized societies" had less painful labor and disputed the idea that only fear made contractions hurt. They also argued that education about childbirth did not eliminate its pain and gave evidence that maternal and infant mortality had decreased because of modern obstetric methods. In short, the authors believed there were no proven psychological benefits of a "natural birth." Although the authors mentioned Read only tangentially, their article refuted each and every point of his fear-tension-pain theory. Even Eastman expressed concern in an editorial appended to a paper by Thoms.[23]

Read's response did not assuage his critics. Publicly, he accused them of not reading or understanding his book. Privately, he raged. To Eastman he wrote: "I was not discouraged by your editorial comments. To be discouraged, fortunately, is not in my makeup; otherwise I certainly would not have continued in this work for thirty years in spite of being ostracized, repeatedly insulted by General Medical Councils and subjected to the other antagonistic activities with which

I have been surrounded. I assure you that I enjoy the asperity and absence of enthusiasm and indeed the absence of comprehension of that section of my senior colleagues who are fossilized, immobilized and very largely devitalized." Read proceeded to excoriate physicians with "vested interests," who opposed him, he said, simply to improve their own social, financial, or professional interests; on occasion similar comments appeared in Read's books and lectures. Personal as well as professional pique may have motivated the letter to Eastman. Read also complained that he had detected only apathy among the obstetricians at Johns Hopkins since his visit in 1947 and that Dr. and Mrs. Eastman had acknowledged neither his house gift nor his "bread and butter letter."[24]

In an era when physicians demanded studies, data, and statistical analysis, Read had none to offer. His quest began just as his colleagues were trying to bring obstetric practice up to the scientific standards of other specialties. Read's approach appeared to undermine their efforts even as maternal and neonatal deaths decreased.

Even more disturbing was Read's emotional, contradictory, and inflammatory style. Sir Eardley Holland, a prominent obstetrician and a longstanding friend, told Read: "I would urge you, though, with respect, to take more thought to win the sympathies of the Profession as distinct from the Public, and give more time and take more trouble in doing so. It is true that Browne and Claye and I happen to be comparatively liberally minded men and to be your professional sympathizers and backers. But you seem to have alienated the sympathies of the rest of the Gynaecological world. Have you even considered that you, yourself, may be to some extent to blame for that state of affairs? You have sometimes tried even me very severely!"[25]

The Public's Response

Regardless of problems with colleagues, Read's tactics and ideas worked with patients. Most women did not care about science, but they did like Read's vision of childbirth and mother love. Letters described problems that they had experienced during past pregnancies and the fear that had grown out of these difficulties, and they thanked Read for giving them the courage to try again. Women also criticized the impersonal care that they received from their own physicians, nurses, and midwives. Even though they had never met him or heard him speak, admirers thanked Read for his interest and concern. Many women explained how anesthesia had been forced on them, preventing them from participating in one of the most important experiences in their life—the birth of their child. Read responded personally to each letter.

Books published during between 1930 and 1950 express many of the same ideas found in the letters written to Read. In *The Good Earth*, Pearl Buck describes a Chinese peasant cheerfully returning to work in a rice paddy immediately after a delivery. The scene bears an uncanny resemblance to Read's experience with Flemish and Greek women during World War I. Other novelists disparaged the impersonal care associated with Western obstetric practices. Doris Lessing's novel *A Proper Marriage* includes a long scene in a delivery suite in which the heroine encounters strict and inflexible rules, isolation from friends and family, and an indifferent, if not hostile, medical staff. The heroine finally obtains help, and some relief from suffering, from a native African charwoman—emphasizing once again the benefits to be derived from a natural birth. Mary McCarthy's book *The Group* also highlights the rigidity of medical childbirth practices during the 1930s. In Sylvia Plath's novel *The Bell Jar* the heroine criticizes Twilight Sleep. Observing a delivery with her boyfriend, a medical student, she describes the delivery bed as "some awful torture table, with metal stirrups sticking up in mid-air and all sorts of instruments and wires and tubes." When she learns that Twilight Sleep will obliterate the patient's memory of the painful delivery, she quips that it sounds "like just the sort of drug a man would invent." Considering the resistance to Twilight Sleep among physicians, mostly male, just a few years earlier, Plath's comment is unfair, but it does illustrate the attitude of the public during the time that Read was promulgating his message.[26]

As interest in natural childbirth increased, women sought more information.[27] A meeting reported in *Wife and Citizen: A Journal Advancing the Economic and Social Emancipation of All Women* (1945) illustrates the change. Invited speakers included the physicians R. J. Minnitt and John Elam and Lady Rhys-Williams of the National Birthday Trust Fund. The panel was surprised that "some members of the audience were enthusiastic to the point of heckling the platform that a treatment of relaxation, practiced with some success by a few doctors, was superior to the gas and air analgesia."

Within twelve years of the publication of his first book, Read had garnered support from a vocal and assertive segment of the public. At this point in his campaign, Read received unexpected help from two improbable allies, Fernand Lamaze and the pope.

Fernand Lamaze and the Pope

Russian claims of a method of Pavlovian training that achieved "painless childbirth" for 90 percent of all women intrigued Fernand Lamaze. An obstetrician on the staff of the

Metal Workers Union Hospital in Paris, Lamaze traveled twice to Leningrad to learn more. *Painless Childbirth,* a book describing what he learned, appeared in 1956. It credits Russian psychologists and physicians for both the theory and the practice of painless childbirth. Lamaze gave no credit to Read and even criticized his methods as vague, mystical, and unscientific. In fairness, Lamaze probably had not read Read's book carefully, for he says that the obstetrician from "Birmingham" (Read had practiced in Woking) had had little impact on obstetrics (by 1956 Read's book had been discussed extensively in many countries), had been abused and shunned by the Anglican church (not true), and had not had any new ideas in more than twenty years (partially true). His own method, Lamaze claimed, had none of the shortcomings of Read's. The book by Lamaze, an almost identical book by his assistant Pierre Vellay, and a third by the American writer Marjorie Karmel sparked intense interest. Apparently the public found the "painless" childbirth promised by Lamaze more appealing than the "natural" childbirth promised by Read.[28]

Read quickly responded to all the allegations. Forgetting the nineteenth-century advocates of natural birth whom he had once cited, Read claimed sole authorship of the idea. Privately he criticized the Russians for having "adopted as their own, this obstetric procedure and deformed it by adding a few distractive and dramatic clinical features which in no way alter the basic principles of the 'new discovery' which was published in England twenty-five years previously." In an unpublished paper, Read's response was more caustic. "Lamaze deserves better than this book. It has been said the 'gypsies used to disfigure the child and call it their own.' This book is an unworthy memorial to a man whose intentions were good, but undesirable tactics will taint the noblest design." Since the communists had seized control of Russia, he noted, they had claimed credit for every major innovation in the world, including the works of Shakespeare and Marconi. Read was not surprised, therefore, that they had claimed his idea, too. Perceiving a slight to his country as well as to himself, Read began to call his technique the "English" or "British" method and began to hyphenate his middle and last name. In the end, the feud between Read and Lamaze may have done more to increase public interest in natural childbirth than the books of either protagonist.[29]

Sensing in the fracas moral and spiritual issues that transcended the pride and honor of individuals and nations, Pope Pius XII delivered a special address in 1956 about the moral and spiritual values of natural childbirth. The text, published in its entirety in the *New York Times*, noted that some patients and physicians still believed that the alleviation of childbirth pain, by whatever means, might contravene divine intent. Although childbirth pain might have spiritual value, the pope explained, nothing in the tradition of the Catholic church prohibited human beings from using appropriate methods to alleviate pain. Although he did not judge the relative merits of the "English" or the "Russian" methods, the pope did caution against allowing a fascination with either method to supplant the spiritual values that should accompany every delivery. To the extent that the English method might be less "materialistic," he believed that it might be preferable.[30]

Newspapers around the world responded with bold headlines: "Pope Okays Drugless Childbirth," "Pontiff Approves System of Painless Childbirth," and "Russian Method Is Acceptable for Catholic Mothers." If it rankled Read that headlines read "painless" and "Russian" instead of "natural" and "English," he did not say so, pleased, as he must have been, with the publicity that followed the pope's address. In numerous interviews Read spoke as though the pope had addressed Read's work alone. The silence of the medical establishment during these events bothered his wife, however: "It is a disgrace to England that the pope should be the first to recognize my husband." Presumably she meant "recognize my husband's work."[31]

Concerned though the pope was that physicians should practice "Christian Obstetrics," he must have overlooked portions of Read's book that blamed the church for the pain and complications of modern childbirth. For his part, Read must have overlooked the pope's comment that "painless childbirth, considered as a general fact, is in clear contrast with common human experience today, as well as in the past, even from the earliest times as far as historical sources permit the fact to be verified. The pains of women in childbirth were proverbial . . . and literature, both profane and religious, furnishes proof of this fact."[32] The statement, of course, contradicts Read's premise that once there was a time when primitive women delivered babies easily, safely, and without pain. Philosophical differences, important though they seem, did not deter the pope from awarding, nor Read from accepting, a silver medal for his work. The world press made much of this event, too.

The pope's address and medal were only two of several newsworthy events that happened to Read in 1956. Read issued a record album of the sounds of natural childbirth, with instructions on the jacket. The British Broadcasting Corporation aired a film showing Read delivering a baby, the first televised human birth in the United Kingdom, if not the world. The show was preceded and followed by an appropriate flurry of newspaper articles and interviews. In 1957 Read's English publisher, Heinemann, released a biography of Read, *Doctor Courageous,* by A. Noyes Thomas.[33] Read contributed directly to the text, which has the romantic, sentimental, and apocryphal style of many of his other books. In 1958, at the peak of his influence and fame, Read undertook a second, extensive speaking tour in the United States. A year later he died.

Read was a romantic, a visionary, and a dedicated man, but he was also an anachronism. His message was good and appropriate. Obstetric practice had become impersonal and meddlesome, and it took a person of Read's talents to redirect the attention of the public and physicians to older values, some of which had been lost in the rush to improve obstetric practices and patient safety. This aspect of Read's work puts him in league with Charles Delucina Meigs, the nineteenth-century American obstetrician who argued so long and hard with James Young Simpson about the routine use of anesthesia for vaginal delivery.

Read failed with his colleagues largely because of his style. He relied on rhetoric and emotion, an accepted approach during the nineteenth century but not in the twentieth. A description of Simpson written a century earlier could apply just as well to Read: "In the advocacy or defense of new methods of treatment or of new remedies, he seldom took into account the prejudices, or even the honest convictions, of others. It was enough for him, if what he proposed seemed to himself good for his patients and defensible in science. The physician is for the patient and the good of the patient must be his first and only care. But in reaching [this point] he often trampled on the long cherished convictions of professional brethren, and in consequence made many enemies."[34]

Scientific support for Read's ideas came only after his death. We now know that women who are anxious about labor have high blood levels of adrenaline, longer labors, and an increased incidence of operative deliveries and that simple methods that alleviate anxiety facilitate deliveries and decrease the frequency of some postpartum problems.[35] None of these facts would have surprised Read, but, then, they probably would not have surprised many of the obstetricians who opposed him, either.

The person who best summarized Read's career is Frank Slaughter, the American surgeon and novelist. Reviewing Read's biography, Slaughter wrote: "After it was announced, the Read method was taken up as a sort of cult with considerable mumbo-jumbo and much popular discussion. For some of the official medical opposition to his theories, Read was himself responsible. He advocated principles of relaxation akin to yoga, which he had learned from an Indian noncommissioned officer in World War I. The methods were effective but such an approach spelled quackery to a suspicious medical profession. It illustrates a very important truth: that those who would get rid of existing shibboleths must be careful how they go about it, lest the opposition they create keep the truth from being widely known."[36]

Read's ability to gather support for natural childbirth is significant for two reasons. First, it signified a decline in public faith in the ability of medicine to abolish disease and of anesthesia to dispel pain. The naive proclamations that followed the introduction of surgical anesthesia in 1846 could only breed disillusionment as the limits of medicine and anesthesia became as apparent to the public as it soon did to physicians. What is remarkable is that public optimism lasted long enough to sustain the campaigns of the National Twilight Sleep Association and the National Birthday Trust.

Second, Read couched his campaign for natural childbirth in many of the idioms of traditional theology. He removed from childbirth the stigma of Eve by telling women that childbirth was natural and beautiful, but he also spoke effusively of the role of motherhood in the creation of a better society and a brighter future, all the product of a childbirth without fear. The public would once again discover the social value of pain; the next time its value would be couched in terms borrowed from psychology rather than religious tracts.

PART III

In the Delivery Room

Physicians and Women Together

"Pain Makes Things Valuable"

The Danger of Drugs and the Social Value of Pain

Through the medical careers of most of us, until recent years,

public opinion has demanded that relief of pain be given,

preferably by production of complete amnesia. The doctor

who has refused to give drugs has lost patients because the

only interest a patient has in labour is in the amount of pain

she suffers. She is not interested in the obstetric abnormalities

except insofar as they affect her pain. . . . Finally, we are now in

a third era when public opinion has swung to the feeling that

labour, be it painful or painless, is best conducted without these pain relieving drugs. There are women today who, even if

they have really severe labour pain, knowing of the slight risk of

drugs, are willing to have a natural childbirth. . . . Natural

childbirth, then, is the fashion of today as was the use of

hyoscine [scopolamine] fifteen years ago. If any doctor casts

it out as being unworkable, he will be the loser, because

natural childbirth patients are usually the most intelligent

and grateful patients in one's practice.

—G. H. Hall, in the *Medical Journal of Australia,* 1954

It had taken years for obstetricians to lose their distrust of anesthesia. Once they did, they used ever-increasing amounts of drugs to control the pain of labor. One technique that became popular in the 1930s involved injection of magnesium sulfate (a depressant of the central nervous system) and morphine followed by an enema of ether dissolved in petroleum oil.[1] Not satisfied with the effects of this combination, some physicians added spinal or general anesthesia. Advocates avowed that the method had no detrimental effects on labor or on the well-being of the child—an extraordinary claim considering the large number and large dosages of drugs. Fortunately, few women received such treatment, because most deliveries were still performed by family practitioners and midwives, both of whom seldom used anesthesia. Nevertheless, the philosophy, if not the reality, of practice had changed. By 1950 obstetric anesthesia was in vogue with both physicians and the public.

The trend toward more liberal use of drugs soon aroused concern. Improvements in maternal care had left obstetricians free to focus their attention on the child, and they began to worry about the effects of drugs on the fetus. Patients became concerned when they, too, recognized the dangers. Women asked if freedom from labor pain justified the risks of anesthesia.

Even as concern for the effects of drugs increased, the public reexamined the significance of pain. In a reversal of the social attitudes that had prevailed through much of the nineteenth century, people came to suspect that pain and suffering had purpose and that the abolition of all pain, even during childbirth, might be disadvantageous to the individual and to society. Read's gospel of natural childbirth brought many of these issues into focus.

The Public's Perception of Drugs

Long before Grantly Dick Read had popularized natural childbirth, physicians had been concerned about the effect of drugs on the newborn, particularly with regard to respiration. In 1842 John Snow remarked how physiologists had "amused themselves" by speculating about the mechanisms that initiate sustained breathing at birth. Soon after he started to use anesthesia for obstetric patients, Snow recognized how easily drugs administered to the mother could disrupt the respiratory efforts of the child. Infants delivered from women who had received chloroform, he wrote, did not "kick and scream in the violent way and grasp the bedclothes with the force, during the first minute after birth, that is often observed under other circumstances." By 1930 pharmacologists had described the extraordinary sensitivity of the respiratory mechanisms of the newborn to many of the drugs normally used to relieve labor pain.[2]

Years passed before studies of physiologists and pharmacologists had any substantive influence on medical practice. The turning point came in 1953, when an American anesthesiologist, Virginia Apgar, devised a simple but effective way of evaluating the neonate. Apgar, who was chief of anesthesia at Presbyterian Hospital in New York, developed a scoring system—based on observations of respiratory effort, heart rate, skin color, reflex irritability, and crying—to identify neonates who required resuscitation. She showed that scores varied in relation to the drugs used to anesthetize women for caesarean section. Infants had better (higher) scores when their mothers had spinal anesthesia, presumably because general anesthesia exposed infants to larger amounts of depressant drugs. Thus, Apgar confirmed Snow's observation from 1847 and Zweifel's work from 1876, showing that drugs do cross

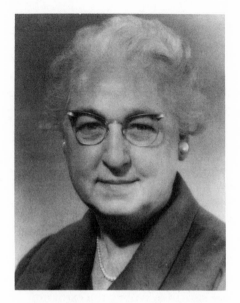

Virginia Apgar (1909–1974). Courtesy
of the Wood Library-Museum of
Anesthesiology, Chicago.

the placenta and that the amounts of anesthetic transferred
were sufficient to affect the child. Her papers raised medical issues dormant since the debate between Simpson and
Meigs one hundred years before.[3]

Other physicians became concerned when they observed an association between low Apgar scores, neonatal
asphyxia, and cerebral palsy. They assumed that the relations
among these variables indicated causality—that asphyxia
during birth caused cerebral palsy later in life and that low
Apgar scores at birth were de facto evidence of prenatal
asphyxia and neurologic damage.[4] Because they knew that
anesthesia could cause lower Apgar scores, physicians also
assumed that anesthesia caused asphyxia in the fetus and

increased risks of permanent neurologic damage. The emphasis on asphyxia as a cause of perinatal disease was the product of a long series of experimental data from physiology laboratories.

Physiologists had been interested in fetal oxygenation even longer than clinicians. As early as the seventeenth century John Mayow had suggested that a major function of the placenta was to facilitate transfer of nitro-aerial particles from the mother to the child. The discovery of oxygen and carbon dioxide early in the nineteenth century stimulated more interest. Soon thereafter, physiologists made crude estimates of the amount of oxygen that a fetus needed to survive and grow. By 1940 they had even measured the amounts of oxygen normally contained in maternal and fetal blood circulating on either side of the placenta.[5]

Physiologic data available in 1953 painted a grim picture of intrauterine life. When Apgar published her first paper, clinicians believed that the fetus developed in a hostile environment, the effect of an imbalance between oxygen supply and demand. They knew that the fetus needed oxygen and that the amounts it needed varied in direct proportion to its size. They believed, however, that the capacity of the placenta to supply oxygen did not increase in proportion to fetal demands. The imbalance between supply and demand was thought to be the cause of many common clinical problems, such as neonatal jaundice and sudden death in utero.

An influential proponent of this theory was Sir Joseph Barcroft, professor of physiology at Cambridge University and author of one of the first authoritative books on prenatal life. Barcroft thought the supply of oxygen at term was so tenuous that only the onset of labor spared the child an asphyxial death in utero. His opinion influenced clinicians, who already knew that labor itself imposed significant stress. Early radiographic studies showed that each contraction of the uterus slowed, if it did not stop, the flow of blood through the placenta, thereby threatening an already marginal oxygen supply. Anesthesia, clinicians believed, diminished oxygen stores even further, adding additional stress.[6] To obstetricians, these data suggested that every delivery, even the most normal, threatened the child with serious injury or death.

The influence of physiology on obstetrics merits comment. Throughout the nineteenth century, French and German physicians worked to apply scientific methods to medical practice. Developments in obstetrics attest to their success. In 1840 obstetric practice was virtually indistinguishable from midwifery. The risks for women were high, and clinicians had few good methods to handle common problems. Obstetricians relied on intuition to evaluate new drugs and techniques, and rhetoric to convince others that their opinions were right. This approach satisfied patients and impressed some colleagues but did little to improve obstetric practice. By 1940 medicine had changed. Clinical studies and laboratory experiments had become accepted ways to evaluate innovations, and obstetrics consequently improved. By 1950 the maternal death rate in the United States had decreased to one-eighth that in 1870 and to one-fourth that in 1900. The health of the newborns had also improved.[7]

Basing obstetric practice on science did not preclude error. Indeed, the use of Apgar scores and physiologic data led obstetricians astray, in part through overinterpretation of the data. Scientists had shown that asphyxia could damage the fetal brain, but assuming that asphyxia was the primary cause of cerebral palsy caused them to overlook other possibilities. Cerebral palsy might simply predispose the child to asphyxia during labor, for instance. Likewise, they knew that severe asphyxia could predispose the neonate to low Apgar scores—scientists had established that in the laboratory. Yet there were no data to support the often-made assertion that a low Apgar score was prima facie evidence of prior asphyxia. Even the physiologic data, which had once seemed so definitive, proved misleading. Investigators found that the deterioration in fetal oxygenation reported by Barcroft was an artifact of his experiments rather than a true measure of placental insufficiency.[8] Later work would correct all these errors, but not before they influenced clinical practice.

There was one important difference between the new debates about obstetric anesthesia and the old: for the first time, the public understood the medical issues. Although the public may not have grasped the complexities of physiologic experiments or the significance of the clinical studies, they did recognize the potential for drug damage and the need for caution. This understanding had been absent from the debates about obstetric anesthesia in 1847, when Simpson first suggested the idea, in 1914, when Twilight Sleep was debated, and even in 1940, when Grantly Dick Read sparred with leaders of the National Birthday Trust Fund.

Virginia Apgar deserves considerable credit for educating the public. An enthusiastic, articulate, and engaging person, reporters sought her out and publicized her work. "Apgar score" became a household phrase. Apgar created even more interest in fetal drug effects after she left her post at the College of Physicians and Surgeons at Columbia University to become director of the Section on Congenital Defects of the National Foundation, March of Dimes. There she helped to make the health of women and newborn children matters of public policy.[9]

Not just Apgar's work but other developments focused

public attention on the potential for drug damage during pregnancy. Two tragedies were especially important. The first involved diethylstilbestrol, an artificial form of estrogen once given to women who had a high incidence of spontaneous abortions. Several years after that practice had stopped, epidemiologists reported an unusually high frequency of genital tumors among daughters of women who had received the drug during pregnancy, presumably an effect of exposure to the hormone at some critical stage of embryonic development. Equally disturbing were reports of severe limb deformities among children whose mothers had taken thalidomide, a sedative once given during early pregnancy.

Other discoveries were less sensational in outcome but equally important in shaping public opinion. Women learned that cigarettes and alcohol increased the risk of damage to the child. Growing publicity associated with the environmental movement caused more concern. Rachel Carson's book *Silent Spring* shocked the public with descriptions of reproductive complications among populations of animals exposed to minute amounts of pesticides. Psychologists and pediatricians found that exposure to minimal amounts of anesthetics altered newborn feeding patterns. They also suggested that anesthesia altered the social interactions between the newborn child and its mother, a subtle effect not detectable with conventional clinical methods and apparent only to highly trained observers. Because these results were unexpected and occurred with forms of anesthesia originally thought to be innocuous, the data worried physicians.[10] As women learned about more of these problems through articles in newspapers and magazines, they asked sharper questions about obstetric anesthesia and looked more favorably toward natural childbirth.

The Public's Perception of Medicine

Adverse publicity about drugs accounts for only part of the growing distrust of obstetric anesthesia. Ironically, patients became concerned when most of the danger had passed —after obstetricians had had a century of experience with anesthesia, most of it good—and when the risks had been reduced by the introduction of better drugs and new techniques.

To a large extent, the increasing distrust of obstetric anesthesia marked a change in the public's perception of risk in general. Social pressure demanded formulation of a new calculus of suffering. By 1950 patients were far more skeptical and cautious about medical innovations than they had been during most of the nineteenth century.[11] This distrust was not limited to anesthesia, nor even to medicine, but was increasingly apparent in many areas of life. The sociologist Robert Nisbet has suggested that the public had lost its faith in the idea of progress by the early decades of the twentieth century.

Nisbet defines the idea of progress as a belief that the course of Western civilization consists of progressive improvement in the political, intellectual, and material aspects of life.[12] Faith in progress, he suggests, stimulated many of the remarkable accomplishments of the nineteenth century —the industrial revolution, social and political reforms, and the migration of foreigners to the Americas and to the American West. Excited by a pervasive atmosphere of optimism, people embraced new ideas, traveled to unexplored areas of the earth, and used new technology with reckless disregard for the consequences. Science and technology could permanently improve the well-being of humankind, it was certain, and any problems that arose could quickly be resolved. In this context, the enthusiasm of women for obstetric anesthesia is simply one manifestation of a philosophy that permeated society. As faith in progress waned, pessimism replaced optimism, and the public became more cautious and fearful, especially about technology. Naturally enough, women became more skeptical about anesthesia, too.

According to Nisbet, pessimism arose during the nineteenth century among a small group of intellectuals, among them Nietzsche, who wrote, "One must go forward step by step into further decadence," and Henry Adams, who predicted "ultimate, colossal, cosmic collapse." Burckhardt, Spengler, and Weber expressed similar ideas. Pessimism increased after the devastation of World War I, accompanied by gloomy pronouncements from the historian J. B. Bury, the church cleric W. R. Inge—who once called progress a "pernicious superstition"—and influential poets, such as William Butler Yeats and T. S. Eliot. According to Nisbet, each of these men attacked tenets that were essential for faith in progress:

(a) A belief in the value of the past,
(b) A conviction of the nobility, even superiority, of Western civilization,
(c) An acceptance of the worth of economic and technological growth,
(d) A faith in reason and in the kind of scientific and scholarly knowledge that can come from reason alone, and
(e) A belief in the intrinsic importance, the ineffaceable worth of life on this earth.

The pessimism that began among a handful of intellectuals gradually spread among other strata of society.

Grantly Dick Read's ideas fit Nisbet's thesis quite well. Read challenged the superiority of Western civilization, maintaining that Judeo-Christian values had created more problems for childbirth than they had solved. Read also criticized technology, suggesting that modern obstetric techniques had damaged more women and children than they had helped. Read trusted intuition more than science, to the point that he ridiculed physicians who used scientific methods to improve practice. He described a world of "misery, privation, bereavement, torture of mind and body, destruction of souls . . . a world swayed by the acquisition of wealth and domination."[13] His faith in mother love was his one expression of optimism. For him, it signified the only force that could restore the world to better order.

Read's crusade coincided with a similar movement in pediatrics. In 1945, the year after Read published the first American edition of his book *Motherhood in the Post War World,* Benjamin Spock published *The Common Sense Book of Baby and Child Care.*[14] There are similarities between the two. Like Read, Spock reassured parents of the superiority of innate knowledge ("You know more than you think you do") and advised women not to be "overawed by what the experts say." Like Read, he challenged the authority of medical science, and his book sold well.

The Social Value of Pain and Suffering

During the many centuries when people had been unable to abolish pain, they had learned to use it and, eventually, to depend on it—to maintain order and to collect information. Courts tortured heretics and maimed criminals. Political leaders made threats of pain and death to mobilize communities and to create a sense of common purpose. At least as far back as biblical times, educators found pain an effective way of promoting learning; with only slight modification, generations of pedagogues taught that we must, as the Book of Proverbs says, "suffer unto truth." Sacrificial pain, a concept so important in the development of early Christian theology, influenced many spheres of life. The church canonized, poets eulogized, and politicians decorated those who endured pain or risked death for the common good. Depictions of pain and martyrdom became favorite themes in art, literature, and music. When nineteenth-century reformers tried to eliminate pain from human experience, they disrupted many important Western cultural traditions.[15] Eventually this inconsistency had repercussions.

Nineteenth-century intellectuals recognized the conundrum: the absence of pain and suffering threatened to produce social chaos. In effect, early social engineers found themselves facing questions similar to those confronting the physicians who first used anesthesia: Is it safe to abolish pain and suffering? How much pain and suffering are necessary to make society work? Physicians resolved their dilemma rather quickly. Within a year they had made anesthesia and the relief of pain hallmarks of modern medicine. Social engineers had considerably more difficulty; they are arguing the merits of suffering even to this day.

Manifestations of the public's ambivalence toward suffering appeared early, as in nineteenth-century parliamentary debates about social reform. Though highly motivated to develop welfare programs for England's poor, politicians thought that some people would not work unless threatened by hunger or pain. Accordingly, they argued how they might distinguish the "earnest" or "deserving poor," those who would benefit from welfare programs, from the "undeserving poor," those who would accept aid indefinitely without attempting to become independent. Similar debates occurred among humanists who wished to reform England's penal codes. They believed that the goal of the penal system should be rehabilitation, not punishment, but they also recognized that social order would disintegrate unless the law retained its authority to punish, with pain if necessary. To meet these dual goals, humanists explored how to administer a "just measure of pain," that is, how to inflict punishment in proportion to the severity of the crime. Gilbert and Sullivan satirized this concept in *The Mikado* when they had the Lord High Executioner sing, "My purpose all sublime, I shall achieve in time, to make the punishment fit the crime." By the end of the nineteenth century most Western countries had abolished corporal punishment, reformed their penal codes, and established the rudiments of welfare programs.

Nor was concern about the social function of pain and suffering confined to parliamentary debates. Writers explored the role of pain as punishment, as a prerequisite for knowledge, and as a sacrifice endured by an individual for the common good. Commenting on early literature, one critic, Northrop Frye, notes how often suffering has characterized larger-than-life tragic figures, such as Prometheus, Hamlet, Faustus, Tamburlaine, and Macbeth.[16]

Many twentieth-century authors have explored the significance of pain and suffering to the society and the individual. In Ernest Hemingway's *The Snows of Kilimanjaro,* the hero is a writer dying of gangrene who recalls how his creativity diminished as his material life improved. Referring to the death of both his creativity and his body, the writer remarks, "The marvelous thing is that it's painless. That's how you know when it starts." Hemingway implies that spiritual and physical death, unlike life, are states free of pain. In real life, Hemingway made the same point to F. Scott Fitzgerald: "You especially have to hurt like hell before you can write seriously. But when you get the damned hurt, use it—

don't cheat with it. Be as faithful to it as a scientist." Richard Wright, in his autobiography, suggests that the true meaning of life emerges only when one struggles "to wring meaning out of meaningless suffering." Walker Percy deals often with suffering in his novels. In *Love in the Ruins* he describes a woman who is terrified by the emptiness of a life without pain, a "well-nigh perfect life, really death in life, in Paradise, where all her needs were satisfied and all she had to do was play golf and bridge." In *The Moviegoer* Percy creates a character who welcomes accidents and personal tragedies as a means to escape the "pain of malaise." As Wallace Stegner succinctly writes, "Pain makes things valuable." In effect, each author poses some variation of the questions asked by the nineteenth-century physicians who confronted the use of anesthesia: "Is there life without pain? What happens to life when we abolish pain?"[17]

Other authors directly address the tension that may develop when a society simultaneously attempts to abolish pain and preserve it. For example, in *The Power and the Glory*, Graham Greene contrasts the moral and spiritual suffering of a timid priest who sacrifices his life for his parishioners to the physical pain of his adversary, a police lieutenant with a toothache. To the priest, pain and suffering are unavoidable, if not necessary, parts of life: "Joy always depends on pain. Pain is part of joy. This is why I tell you that heaven is here: this is a part of heaven just as pain is part of heaven." The police lieutenant, on the other hand, utters comments typical of nineteenth-century social reformers: "We'll give people food, teach them to read, give them books. We'll see they don't suffer. Suffering is wrong." The priest dies a martyr and the lieutenant lives with his toothache, leaving the reader to ponder which man won and which man knew the truth.[18]

Wallace Stegner compares different philosophies of pain in *All the Little Live Things*. Stegner's main character, an older man who is embittered by the premature death of his only son, says, "Pain is fine when you can turn it off. It may even be good for the soul in small quantities [but] pain is poison. Don't go hunting for it. . . . Avoid it all you can and bear it if you must, but never mistake it for something desirable!" Another character, a pregnant woman dying of breast cancer, counters: "How would women feel if having babies was as easy as picking apples? Don't you get pleasure—satisfaction—no, pleasure it really is—out of all the rough, hot, cold, scratchy, hard uncomfortable things?" Convinced that pain must be accepted if one is to live fully, she is determined to give birth and to die without drugs. That Stegner uses childbirth to illustrate his point, and that he compares painless childbirth to picking apples, is especially pertinent in the context of this discussion.[19]

In Stegner's book the dying woman's ordeal serves as a nidus for the formation of a social unit. The story highlights both the communal nature of childbirth and role of suffering as a mechanism for the formation of a social bond. This, too, is pertinent, because much of the current dissatisfaction with obstetrics derives in part from the disruption of the social aspects of childbirth brought about by anesthesia and other technical practices.

The Social Conventions of Childbirth

Anesthesia promised a safer, more comfortable delivery, an explicit goal of the technological revolution of the nineteenth century. Yet anesthesia and all the other technological improvements in obstetrics disrupted social conventions. As modern medicine lessened the fear of pain and death in childbirth, it also diminished the importance of two stimuli that had once had served to elicit communal support. As deliveries moved from homes to hospitals, nurses and social workers performed functions that once had been the responsibility of neighbors, and obstetricians displaced midwives. All that remained of the rich cultural, social, and religious traditions surrounding childbirth were the ritual baby showers and gifts of diapers and baby formula donated by commercial vendors. Women were healthier and lived longer, but childbirth had become technical and impersonal.

These changes were not unique to obstetrics. In the twentieth century the technical aspects of hospital care have become increasingly important for all branches of medicine. Hospitals are highly regimented and paternalistic not only by necessity but also by tradition. The historian Charles Rosenberg suggests that these characteristics arose in early hospitals, founded by religious orders, which were as concerned about the moral improvement of their patients as about the treatment of disease. Paternalism, Rosenberg believes, was a method later used in nursing and other professions to gain professional identity.[20]

But patients disliked the isolation and impersonal care in hospitals. Even as various organizations were campaigning to increase the availability of obstetric beds in British hospitals, women were complaining about the nature of the care. In a survey conducted in 1948 by the Royal College of Obstetricians and Gynaecologists, half of the fifteen thousand women interviewed "preferred" delivery within their own home, which, in reality, meant care by a midwife without anesthesia. Their reasons are pertinent. Four percent felt safer at home, but another 8 percent simply wanted to remain near their family. It was the impersonal, if not calloused, nature of hospital deliveries that Doris Lessing portrayed in her novel *A Proper Marriage*.[21] Natural childbirth, Lamaze training, childbirth education, and related movements all became part of the reaction against these modern obstetric methods.

Two recent historical studies give more insight into early social conventions surrounding childbirth, including the role of pain and suffering. In the first study, *A Midwife's Tale*, the author, L. T. Ulrich, uses the diary of Martha Ballard, a midwife, to reconstruct life in a small rural community in Maine. During the thirty-year period between the Revolutionary War and the War of 1812 Ballard delivered more than eight hundred babies, losing only four mothers, a very commendable record for that time and place.[22]

Because of the distance and poor roads, women usually called Ballard early to their homes. While waiting for labor to begin, she helped with household chores. With the onset of active labor, neighbors also came to help. After the delivery all joined in a celebratory dinner. Ulrich notes that Ballard describes the three stages of labor not in biological terms, as we would today, but in social terms: first, the arrival of the midwife; next, of neighbors; and, finally, of an afternurse to assist the woman during recovery.

Ballard seldom mentions pain in her diary, although she does use euphemisms such as "illness." To the women of Martha Ballard's community, as to Anne Bradstreet a century earlier, childbirth meant pain and the real possibility of death. Neighbors responded by helping the woman and caring for her family. Ulrich suggests that the social bonds forged during this experience lasted long after the delivery itself.

Another study describes social functions of childbirth pain among the English aristocracy. To learn the attitudes of this group, J. S. Lewis reviewed diaries and letters written by fifty women between 1760 and 1860. Lewis found out that childbirth pain helped establish a woman's position within her family. The aristocratic wife was responsible for producing the male heir. The manner in which she faced childbirth and its pain and danger became a measure of her character and of her sacrifice. Through the experience she earned status and personal security, in the same way that her husband earned social approval through his performance on the battlefield.[23]

Ancient Greeks, too, likened childbirth to battle, and wounds to labor pain. In Euripides' play *Medea* the lead character says: "They say that we have a safe life at home, whereas men must go to war. Nonsense! I had rather fight three battles than bear one child." Homer, too, compared war wounds with labor pain:

> But soon as the gash dried and firm clots formed,
> sharp pain came bursting in on Atrides' strength—
> agonies brought on by the harsh, birthing spirits,
> Hera's daughters who hold the stabbing power of
>   birth—
> so sharp the throes that burst on Atrides' strength.

Similarly, Spartans accorded high status to the pain of childbirth. Their tombs commemorated only two types of death: from battle and from childbirth.[24]

Thus, in several cultures the pain of childbirth, however unpleasant for the individual, served as a mechanism to forge and maintain social bonds. Ironically, the medical discoveries that increased the comfort and safety of women may have inadvertently disrupted important social patterns.

The Medical Response

Obstetric practice changed in response to public pressure to restore some of the social and family connotations of childbirth. Obstetricians first allowed and then encouraged family participation in childbirth. Husbands, relatives, or friends accompanied women to educational classes to learn how to give physical and emotional support during labor. Although these methods were initially praised for their psychological benefits, subsequent studies revealed medical advantages as well. Women who had the company of a supportive person during labor were less likely to have a prolonged labor and less likely to need a forceps delivery or caesarean section than women who had no support.[25]

Clinicians eventually found physiologic explanations for these phenomena. Emotional support seemed to lessen fear and hence the blood concentration of hormones normally released by the body during stress—the catecholamines. The ability of catecholamines to slow or stop labor provides a mechanism for animals to slow or stop labor if danger threatens, but it produces a dysfunctional effect in the woman in labor who is stressed only by fear. One study has suggested that emotional support during labor even decreases the incidence of postpartum depression. Grantly Dick Read had predicted that reducing fear would have obstetric benefits. He had based his opinion on intuition, and correct or not, intuitive assertions were not sufficient to convince a generation of physicians who had been trained to verify theory by experimentation.

Soon after fathers and families again became part of the birthing process, there appeared a group of paraprofessionals called "doulas," "birth partners," or "professional birth assistants." They modeled their role after the work of lay midwives in third world countries, who assist women in labor and who often also provide prenatal and postnatal counseling. In the United States virtually all of these practitioners are women. Their training and medical knowledge varies: some have considerable experience as midwives or nurses; others are laypeople whose primary qualification is their own experience with labor; yet others may just want to help. All charge for their services.[26]

The role of doulas is somewhat ambiguous. They are part of the movement to place childbirth back in a traditional social context. In this regard, they, like Grantly Dick Read, endorse the importance of the birth experience to the emotional and psychological development of the mother and child. They argue that nurses and physicians cannot satisfy the psychological and physical needs of women in labor. Although doulas do not reject the use of anesthesia and modern obstetric techniques, they tend to discourage them.

The beliefs of doulas contradict some of the ideas that once characterized the natural childbirth movement. Even though doulas encourage the participation of the father, for example, they argue that a man cannot give a woman the support she needs. They believe that the best help comes when women help women, but it is even better, they say, when such help comes from a doula rather than the patient's mother, aunt, sister, or nurse. They wish to serve the patient as a friend or family member would, yet they charge a fee. Doulas have no medical credentials or legal responsibilities, but often they advocate one mode of obstetric management over another and sometimes suggest measures that contradict accepted medical practice. In effect, they seek to combine the atmosphere of a traditional delivery with the medical advantages and safety of modern obstetrics. In doing so, they have interposed a new layer between the patient and hospital staff.

For childbirth, the first half of the twentieth century was a period of reflection and reevaluation. When the century began, enthusiasm for anesthesia was unbridled. William Osler (1849–1919), one of the era's most famous physicians, wrote: "The desire to take medicine is perhaps the greatest feature which distinguishes man from animals." This changed, not only because women became more sophisticated about drugs and their effects but also because they came to feel differently about risk. People became as afraid of medicine as of disease and, less willing to trust innovation than before, wanted a return to traditional practices.

"The Greatest Misery of Sickness Is Solitude"

Current Controversy

The abdication of Belief

Makes the Behavior small —

Better an *ignis fatuus*

Than no illume at all.

— Emily Dickinson, circa 1882

All of the reactions to the pain of childbirth that I have found in history I have also observed among my patients. Most request anesthesia—this has been the predominant response of women for more than a century. Some refuse. Of these, a small number have a labor that is so short or so easy that they do not need anesthesia. Others refuse because they fear the effects of anesthesia for either themselves or their child. Still others prefer "natural birth," the only method available for centuries and even now the only method available to most women in the world. Rarely, a patient refuses anesthesia for religious reasons, alluding to God's just punishment of Eve and all her descendants.

The response of friends and family also varies. Most people, disturbed by a woman's pain, appear agitated. They may rub her back or hand, or ask the nurse or physician, "Can't you make her more comfortable?" or "Are you sure she is all right?" Sometimes they try to reassure the woman by suggesting that the pain is important or has purpose. Recently I heard a mother tell her daughter, "I know the pain is bad, but this is what makes you love your child afterward. This is why you take care of your baby." I am sure the experience of childbirth that this mother and daughter shared helped build social bonds comparable to those described by the nineteenth-century midwife Martha Ballard.

Other families react in less supportive ways. Occasionally parents may refuse to give permission for their daughter's anesthetic even though she herself has asked for it. One mother told me, "Don't give her anything. I want her to learn something." At first the mother's reaction seemed harsh and cruel. Prompted to elaborate, however, she noted that her fourteen-year-old daughter was unmarried and that she would return to school soon after the delivery. She was angry with her daughter for becoming pregnant and was pessimistic about her future. The mother also knew that she herself would have to raise the child until her daughter completed her education and found a job. To this mother, the pain of childbirth was punishment and a lesson to teach her daughter the implications of parenthood. I suspect, however, that the pain also represented a form of atonement, a method by which the daughter might reestablish her position within the family. Education, punishment, and atonement are all traditional functions of pain.

Families sometimes use the woman's pain to teach others. During labor a parent may turn to their daughter's partner and say, "See what you have done" or "See what she is doing for you." To them, the daughter's pain represents a sacrifice that obligates him to care for the daughter and the child. This use of pain to establish a social contract resembles the use that the historian J. S. Lewis found described in letters and diaries of nineteenth-century English aristocrats.

Very disturbing are social situations in which the woman's ordeal has no discernible effect on those attending her. Sometimes a boyfriend or parent will sit through an entire labor and show no emotion and offer no support. Clearly, simply witnessing a woman's pain, fear, or anguish during childbirth does not guarantee the development of social bonds. Conversely, absence of pain does not mean that social bonds will fail to develop. Most families continue to give their emotional and physical support even after the woman's pain has been relieved with anesthesia. I am sure that the social response to the pain of childbirth depends in large part on the character and strength of the relationships that exist before labor begins.

No less varied are the reactions of physicians and nurses. Many nurses with whom I worked thirty years ago distrusted anesthesia. They had learned effective methods to help women through childbirth without anesthesia simply because it was not available. Like many nineteenth-century physicians who objected to anesthesia, these nurses thought anesthesia unsafe. Today such reactions are rare. Most nurses believe that anesthesia is safe, and urge it on their patients out of compassion or because they believe it to be medically advantageous.

Even among contemporary nurses, however, reactions may vary. Recently I overheard one nurse tell another, "With my next pregnancy I want an epidural anesthetic at seven months." By this she meant that she expected to be physically uncomfortable throughout the last trimester of pregnancy and, like the heroine in Edith Wharton's novel *Twilight Sleep*, preferred to avoid the whole experience. The other nurse responded, "I had both my babies without any anesthesia. It was very hard, but I think that it made me a better person." The two nurses are similar in age, experience, and training. Having worked with each of them, I know how differently they handle patients. Patients of the first nurse request anesthesia more often than those of the second, a reflection, I am sure, of the differences in their personal beliefs.

Predictably, physicians also react differently toward the pain of childbirth, although their personal values often are hidden by an overlay of science. Theoretically, medical training should minimize this variation, based as it is on scientific principles and the analysis of clinical trials. Certainly contemporary physicians are better prepared in science than their predecessors were. In fact, however, modern physicians must reconcile very complicated issues, many of which were not even perceived as problems a few generations earlier. When John Snow anesthetized Queen Victoria, for example, physicians measured success in obstetrics by the survival of the mother and perhaps the child. Now both physicians and the public take survival for granted. Instead they worry whether exposure to an anesthetic will affect a newborn's intelligence or personality, how vigorously it will suckle, whether the child is likely to become a drug addict later in life or unlikely to form a strong psychological bond with its parents — to mention just a few contemporary issues. Each problem, complex in itself, must be reassessed with the introduction of every new drug, the modification of any existing drug, or the use of an established drug in a new way. Progress in medical science is slow. Conclusions drawn even from well-designed studies seldom are definitive. Thus, two competent physicians may examine the same data and reach different conclusions about the most appropriate form of pain management. This leaves considerable room for variation in patient care.

Criticism of Modern Practice

Having observed the complex response of patients, families, nurses and physicians to the pain of childbirth, I discount many critics of current practice. These critics say that contemporary methods make childbirth unnecessarily mysterious, that an intimate event once conducted by midwives in the home has now become a highly technical process managed by strangers, albeit professionals, in a hospital. Critics acknowledge that modern practice has brought gains, but they suggest that the frequent use of anesthesia, uterine stimulants, and surgery creates more problems than it solves. They suggest that modern practices disenfranchise women, place them under the control of physicians, foster gender stereotypes, and undermine the social bonds that otherwise might develop among women were they to care for each other in the home. The only women who benefit from modern obstetric practices, they speculate, are those with unusual medical problems.[1]

Some critics impugn the motives of physicians. They suggest that physicians support technical hospital deliveries to enhance their income or to improve their social and professional status. One author writes, "When obstetrics gained political ascendancy in American birthing practices, and births were moved into the hospital, the needs and interests of birthing women were subordinated to the needs and interests of the profession of medicine." Another suggests that "novel technologies represented the tool with which the obstetrician could implement the program of childbirth engineering." Describing the relationship between obstetricians and patients, critics may use such terms as "control," "power," "managed," "negotiation," "manipulation of professional boundaries," "legal monopoly on practice," "shrewd politicking," and "manipulation of the public's view of birth by exploitation of metaphors."[2]

I disagree with these critics for several reasons. First, the transition from midwife to obstetrician, from home to hospital, and from natural childbirth to anesthesia was initiated as much by patients as by physicians. This movement began among feminists in response to the high incidence of problems associated with childbirth. During the nineteenth century, maternal death rates had hardly declined despite substantial improvements in other areas of medicine. Physicians and patients alike believed that childbirth would be safer and women more comfortable if deliveries were in hospitals rather than homes. In this regard, even the movement toward hospitalization for childbirth was part of a larger trend. During the last decades of the nineteenth century, physicians began to rely upon hospitals for management of medical problems as diverse as tuberculosis and insanity. As the historian Charles Rosenberg has observed, the expanding role of hospital care was influenced as much by cultural and political pressures as by any change in the philosophy of medical practice.[3] In fact, obstetrics was among the last of the medical specialties to shift care from home to hospital, to the consternation of social activists and many patients.

Contrary to the comments of critics, developments in science and medicine have done more to demystify obstetrics than to make it more complex. Physicians know far more about the biology of reproduction, anatomy, physiology, and the treatment of pain than ever before. This information is readily available to any curious patient who is willing to ask questions or to read the books and articles prepared for their use.

Words such as *power* and *control* also mislead, particularly when used to describe medical practice. Critics, many of whom are concerned only with social issues, often overlook the medical connotations of the words. To a physician the "power" of an anesthetic may be its ability to keep a patient pain-free and motionless during a caesarean section or a difficult vaginal delivery. In this context, the words do not imply intimidation, subjugation, or force, as they might in a political process. It is noteworthy that the medical procedures that critics find objectionable are the same ones that male physicians choose for their wives and that female physicians choose for themselves.[4]

More important, however, I believe that critics overlook the tremendous variation in the expectations of patients and their families and the difficulty that such variation presents to the nurses and physicians who care for them. Childbirth is a personal, emotional, and physical event, one of great significance to the woman and to members of her social group.

It is virtually impossible to predict how a patient and her family will respond to all these factors, much less how they will interact with nurse and physician.

Consider the problem of the adolescent girl whose family refuses to give permission for her to have an anesthetic for labor. In my community parental permission is not necessary, because a pregnant adolescent is considered an "emancipated minor." As such, she has the legal right to give consent: I may administer an anesthetic despite objections by her parents. Whether it would be wise to ignore the parents is another matter, however. I can relieve the girl's pain, but she and her child must live with the family afterward and depend on them for physical, emotional, and financial support. In such circumstances I wonder about the long-term effects of using the anesthetic. Will their support for the daughter and her child be less if they believe that she has avoided the punishment and the lesson that the pain of childbirth was supposed to offer?

Consider, too, the problem confronting a physician who believes that anesthesia for childbirth has medical benefits. How should this physician temper the advice given to a woman who favors natural childbirth? Similarly, how should a physician handle a patient who demands anesthesia, not because of the pain she is having, but because she fears the pain that she expects to have? Should the physician incur the risks of anesthesia simply because she is afraid? In practice, such problems are not uncommon. Faced with families and patients who are gripped by fear and pain, issues of "power," "control," "childbirth engineering," and "shrewd politicking" never even arise.

Most important, however, I believe that critics have overlooked the great problems posed by pain itself.

The Problem of Pain

The dramatic developments in science and medicine during the nineteenth century, including the introduction of surgical anesthesia, challenged traditional ideas about the nature of pain, as well as the nature of suffering, disease, and death. Physicians learned the importance of dealing with pain as if it were simply a biological process. They identified the types of stimuli that induce pain, the receptors that detect it, the nerves that carry the information to the brain, and the neurologic mechanism that coordinates an appropriate response from the rest of the body. Descriptions of pain by prominent scientists illustrate the extent of change. Writing in 1915, for example, one physician characterized pain as the "representation in consciousness of a change produced in a nerve center by a special mode of excitation . . . a mental state . . . due to the perception of an injury to the body or a feeling." A Nobel Laureate in physiology from the same period called pain the "physical adjunct of an imperative protective reflex."[5] Both scientists made significant contributions to our understanding of the function of the nervous system and the biologic properties of pain.

However beneficial for medicine, divesting pain of its social and religious connotations created both practical and philosophical problems, many of which still confront us today. The practical problem confronting physicians was the mastery of science. When anesthesia first appeared, science was not part of medical practice. The average physician probably knew little more about the biology of disease and pain than many well-read laypeople. Most medical schools had very low academic standards. Many physicians still learned medicine by apprenticeship or by independent reading. In the United States science did not become a required part of medical education until after publication of the Flexner report in 1910.[6] Accordingly, even though the management of pain required scientific study and analysis, few physicians were capable of such work. I suspect that the average physician in 1847 was hardly better prepared to evaluate the effects of anesthesia on childbirth than were many of his patients. Physicians, given their inexperience, were wise to be cautious.

Patients were less cautious. Between 1847 and 1920 most thought that the pain of childbirth was neither natural nor desirable. Moreover, they believed anesthesia to be an unmixed blessing, an example of the ability of science and technology to overcome any adversity. Eager to be free of pain, unaware of the technical problems posed by anesthesia, and unfamiliar with the slow pace of medical progress, many patients thought the delay in using anesthesia for childbirth unconscionable. Public impatience surfaced in 1847, after the introduction of ether and chloroform, and again in 1914, with the appearance of Twilight Sleep. Not until 1940 did American women and physicians reconcile their differences. Ironically, they reached this accord just as public interest was beginning to shift toward natural childbirth. Soon thereafter, medical science and public sentiment were once again out of phase, this time with patients touting the virtues of natural birth and physicians defending the use of drugs.

Though disruptive, the practical problems arising from the clinical use of anesthesia probably had less impact on public satisfaction than did concomitant changes in perceptions of pain. Certainly, perceptions were changing even before the introduction of anesthesia. It does seem likely that the discovery of the anesthetic properties of ether and chloroform accelerated the transition in the approach to pain, from viewing it as a phenomenon with social and religious connotations to studying it as a biological process. As pain and suffering lost their social and religious connotations, however, patients unwittingly lost an important way to cope. Pain's value as a punishment, as a means to learn, as a mechanism to establish and maintain social order, and even as a path to find God had diminished.

Each advance in biology and medical science helped foster the idea that pain is a human experience, one that has no intrinsic meaning. For example, the nineteenth-century poet Emily Dickinson wrote that "Pain—has an Element of Blank"; it is an experience

> Remembered, if outlived
> As Freezing persons, recollect the Snow
> First—chill—then stupor—then the letting go.

Decades later the novelist V. S. Naipaul wrote, "Pleasure and pain—and above all, pain—had no meaning; to possess pain was as meaningless as to chase pleasure." Even C. S. Lewis, a writer deeply concerned with Western religious traditions, dismissed pain as "one of those awkward facts which must be fit into any system." Scientists expressed such ideas, too. One highly respected investigator wrote, "Reflection tells me that I am so far from being able to satisfactorily define pain . . . that the attempt would serve no useful purpose. . . . We have no knowledge of pain beyond that derived from human experience." Contrast these comments with those of two sixteenth-century poets. George Herbert wrote, "Sorrow was all my soul; I scarce believed/Till grief did tell me roundly, that I lived," and John Donne wrote, "Batter my heart, three-personed God . . . That I may rise, and stand."[7] Both poets imply that pain was an experience that gave them life itself. They did not question its function or importance.

By the nineteenth century perceptions of pain, suffering, disease, and death had undergone great change.

I suspect that the transformation of pain into an awkward biologic fact had no significant impact on patients as long as they maintained their faith in science and medicine. Sometime after 1900, however, this faith began to wane. As disillusionment with industrialization increased, patients came to recognize the limits of medicine. Two early twentieth-century literary works illustrate growing awareness of the problems. *The Doctor's Dilemma* by George Bernard Shaw and *Arrowsmith*, the Pulitzer Prize–winning novel by Sinclair Lewis, deal explicitly with the social, medical, and ethical problems that may arise from premature use of a promising new treatment. Faith in the social and religious connotations of pain having already been shaken by the events of the Enlightenment, now the public slowly lost its faith in science, and in medicine as well. Paradoxically, as the ability of medical science to control pain increased, the ability to control suffering appeared to be lost.

The Difference Between Pain and Suffering

The distinction between pain and suffering is important. To a physician, pain is a biological process, the physical response to a noxious stimulus. Suffering, on the other hand, is a psychological process, one that may occur even in the absence of pain. For physicians, the control of pain is a relatively new responsibility. The treatment of suffering, however, is a very old responsibility that physicians share with many other members of the community: family, friends, and clerics, to name a few.

In a recent book, the physician Eric Cassell examines the

nature of suffering. He describes suffering as "the state of severe distress associated with events that threaten the intactness of person." Such threats may be physical or mental, real or imagined. A common characteristic is the tendency of such threats to create feelings of isolation. The sense of isolation may be immediate and apparent, as when a person is confined to bed by an illness or injury, but it may also occur when illness threatens the individual with a life change. Patients may feel alienated from their own past or from their prospects for the future. Simply put, they despair or lose hope. John Updike makes the same point. He observes how pain isolates the afflicted and

> shows us, too, how those around us
> do not and cannot share
> our being.

Four centuries earlier, John Donne made a similar observation: "As *Sickness* is the greatest misery, so the greatest misery of sickness is *solitude*. . . . Solitude is a torment which is not threatened in *hell* itself." Cassell suggests that the treatment of suffering—Donne's "solitude"—is a major problem confronting modern physicians.[8]

Medical studies confirm the effect of suffering on the experience of pain. Most notable is a classic paper by Henry K. Beecher, an anesthesiologist.[9] Beecher studied the narcotic requirements of American soldiers wounded during the Anzio invasion of World War II. He found that these soldiers required less morphine than a comparable group of American civilians who had sustained similar injuries in industrial accidents. Beecher attributed the difference in narcotic requirements to the social connotations of the wounds. To the civilians, injury meant loss of work and pay and social isolation during recuperation. To the soldiers, the wound meant a trip home, a medal, honorable discharge, reunion with friends and family, and possibly a disability pension. In other words, they appeared to suffer less.

Pain, Suffering, and Childbirth

I believe that suffering may lie at the crux of the problems that periodically arise between patients and physicians regarding the management of childbirth. Traditional explanations, whatever their limitations, gave patients assurance that their pain had purpose and meaning. James Young Simpson undermined this support when he insisted that the pain of childbirth was a biological phenomenon devoid of religious or social significance. In effect, Simpson called for an "abdication of belief" of the sort described by Emily Dickinson in her poem. In time, the abdication had precisely the effect that she predicted: it "made the behavior small."

When proposed, Simpson's idea appealed to large segments of society, and I suspect that patients did not appreciate the value of belief or realize the extent of their loss. In time, however, anesthesia did increase the sense of isolation. Unconscious women could not experience the emotional and physical support of friends and family. Hospitalization for childbirth increased the isolation even more. The nineteenth-century physician George Engelmann may have been correct, therefore, when he said that Victorian women suffered more with childbirth than "primitive" women did. I believe that they suffered not from physical deterioration, as Engelmann suggested, but from their loss of so many of the social and religious conventions that had once sustained them. Although some experts may disagree, Beecher's study corroborates this idea.[10]

Nevertheless, I am intrigued by the persistence of traditional connotations of pain. Many of these appear in the responses of my patients despite all the advances of medical science. Childbearing women support themselves and each other by saying that pain can teach, punish, form social bonds, and increase the love of a mother for her child. I suspect that Simpson himself recognized the importance of these ideas and their resilience. Perhaps this explains why he attacked the religious objections to the use of anesthesia for surgery and obstetrics, even though there had been no such objections. A century later, Grantly Dick Read made the same assumption when he blamed the church for opposition to his new method of natural birth.[11]

Such attacks notwithstanding, church officials have always denied opposition to anesthesia or to methods of natural childbirth. I suspect that any resistance has been in the minds of individual patients who imbue pain and suffering with importance.

Having attacked the church, Grantly Dick Read proceeded to organize a secular religion of his own, one that invested childbirth with a whole new set of rituals and traditions. The goal was "motherlove," rather than reenactment of the consequences of original sin. In any case, the effect was similar: investing the pain of childbirth with purpose.

Childbirth is a momentous event. No one wants it to hurt. On the other hand, no one wants to diminish its importance. It is reassuring to realize that patients find ways to preserve the meaning in childbirth even in the absence of pain and suffering.

NOTES

Chapter One
James Young Simpson and the Beginning of Obstetric Anesthesia

1. H. W. Haggard, *Devils, Drugs and Doctors: The Theory of the Science of Healing from Medicine Man to Doctor* (New York: Harper, 1929), p. 1; H. L. Gordon, *Sir James Young Simpson and Chloroform* (London: T. Fisher Unwin, 1897), pp. 56, 1–36, 53; J. A. Shepard, *Simpson and Syme of Edinburgh* (Edinburgh: Livingstone, 1969), pp. 85, 77–102, 85; Letter from Simpson to his brother, dated January 20, 1847, quoted in Shepard, p. 85.

2. All Bible quotations are from the King James version. Homer, *The Iliad*, book 11, translated by R. Lattimore (Chicago: University of Chicago Press, 1962), pp. 11, 269–272; D. Lessing, *A Proper Marriage* (New York: Plume, 1970), p. 144; S. Plath, *The Bell Jar* (New York: Bantam, 1975), p. 53; J. Hemschemeyer, "Giving Birth in Greek," in *Sutured Words: Contemporary Poetry About Medicine,* edited by J. Mukan (Brookline: Aviva Press, 1987), pp. 234–235.

3. B. M. Duncum, *The Development of Inhalation Anaesthesia* (London: Oxford University Press, 1947); "Anesthetic Agents in Midwifery and Surgery," *Boston Medical and Surgical Journal,* January 12, 1847; R. H. Ellis, "The Introduction of Ether Anesthesia to Great Britain," *Anaesthesia,* 1976, 31:766–777; J. Y. Simpson, "On the Inhalation of Sulphuric Ether in the Practice of Midwifery," *Edinburgh Monthly Journal of Medical Science,* March 1847, pp. 721–732.

4. Gordon, pp. 56, 1–36, 53; Shepard, pp. 85, 77–102; W. Hale-

White, *Great Doctors of the Nineteenth Century* (London: Eduard Arnoud, 1935), pp. 143–158.

5. Gordon, pp. 56, 1–36, 53; "James Young Simpson, Obituary," *British Medical Journal,* May 14, 1870, p. 505: "On the post mortem examination the following observations on Sir James Simpson's head were made:—Skull—circumference round by occipital protuberance and below frontal eminences, 22.5 inches;—from ear to ear, 13 inches;—from occipital protuberance to point between superciliary ridges, 13. Brain—weight of entire brain (cerebrum and cerebellum) was 54 ounces; the cerebellum, pons, and the medulla oblongata weighed 5.25 oz." Phrenology was in vogue for much of the nineteenth century, particularly in Edinburgh. According to prevailing theory, the size of the brain was a good measure of intellect, hence the interest in Simpson's brain. For more information see S. Shapin, "Phrenological Knowledge and the Social Structure of Early Nineteenth-Century Edinburgh," *Annals of Science,* 1975, 32:219–243. Also see Chapter 7 for an overview of the development of theories of neurological function.

6. Shepard, pp. 85, 77–102.

7. In this instance, Simpson obtained chloroform from David Waldie, a chemist whose shop was near his home (Gordon, pp. 106–107); J. Y. Simpson, "A New Anaesthetic Agent More Efficient Than Sulphuric Ether," *Lancet,* 1847, 2:549–551.

8. The poem, entitled *Prometheus,* published in *Lancet,* 1870, 1:564, 704, 717, 853, begins as follows:

"Ah me! alas! pain, pain, ever, for-ever!"
So groaned upon his rock that Titan god,
Who by his brave and loving hardihood
Was to weak man of priceless boons the giver,
Which e'en the supreme tyrant could not sever
From us, once given; we owe him in our food
And in our blazing hearth's beatitude;
Yet still his cry was "pain, ever, for-ever!"

Shall we a later, harder doom rehearse?
One came whose art men's dread of art repressed;
Mangled and withering limbs he lulled to rest,

And stingless left the old Semitic curse;
He, too, for these blest gifts did Zeus amerce?
He, too, had vultures tearing at his breast.

9. "James Young Simpson, Obituary."

10. J. D. Mackie, *A History of Scotland* (Middlesex, England: Penguin Books, 1964), pp. 156, 169.

11. G. L. Geison, *Michael Foster and the Cambridge School of Physiology: The Scientific Enterprise in Late Victorian Society,* (Princeton: Princeton University Press, 1978), pp. 1–78; F. N. L. Poynter, "Medical Education in England Since 1600," in *The History of Medical Education,* edited by C. D. O'Malley (Los Angeles: University of California Press, 1970), pp. 235–250.

12. L. R. C. Agnew, "Scottish Medical Education," in *The History of Medical Education,* edited by C. D. O'Malley (Los Angeles: University of California Press, 1970), pp. 251–262; J. Z. Bowers, "The Influence of Edinburgh on American Medicine," in *Medical Education and Medical Care,* edited by G. McLachlan (Oxford: Oxford University Press, 1977), pp. 1–25; I. Loudon, "Medical Practitioners, 1750–1850, and Medical Reform in Britain," in *Medicine in Society,* edited by A. Wear (Cambridge: Cambridge University Press, 1992), pp. 219–248.

13. Agnew, pp. 251–262; M. Kaufman, *American Medical Education: The Formative Years, 1765–1910* (Westport, Conn.: Greenwood Press, 1976), pp. 3–35.

14. D. Caton, "Obstetric Anesthesia: The First Ten Years," *Anesthesiology,* 1970, 33:102–109; A. D. Farr, "Early Opposition to Obstetric Anaesthesia," *Anaesthesia,* 1980, 35:896–907; J. Duffy, "Anglo-American Reaction to Obstetrical Anesthesia," *Bulletin of the History of Medicine,* 1964, 38:32–44.

15. J. Y. Simpson, "The Works of James Young Simpson," in *The Obstetric Memoirs and Contributions of James Young Simpson,* edited by W. O. Priestly and H. R. Storer (Edinburgh: Adam and Charles Black, 1871), pp. 57, 111–112, 199–200.

16. Mackie, pp. 156, 169.

17. "Report of the Edinburgh Royal Maternity Hospital from 1844 to 1846," *Monthly Journal of Medical Science,* November 1848.

18. Simpson, "Works of James Young Simpson," pp. 57, 111–112, 199–200.

19. J. Y. Simpson, "Letter to C. D. Meigs, January 23, 1848," quoted in W. Channing, *A Treatise on Etherization in Childbirth, Illustrated by Five Hundred Eighty-One Cases* (Boston: William Ticknor, 1848).

Chapter Two
The Opposition to Obstetric Anesthesia

1. F. B. Dexter, "Biographical Sketches of the Graduates of Yale College," in *Annals of the College History,* vol. 4 (New York: Henry Holt, 1907), p. 43; W. L. Kingsley, *Yale College—A Sketch of Its History,* vol. 1 (New York: Henry Holt, 1879), p. 109.

2. By a twist of fate, Crawford Long also attended the college, probably at the same time that Charles Meigs was a student there. Long was the Georgia physician who administered ether for surgery in 1842, four years before Morton did. Long is also said to have anesthetized his own wife for childbirth—several years before Simpson used obstetric anesthesia. He did not publicize his accomplishments, however, and has never received the credit given to Morton or Simpson.

3. E. L. Bauer, *Doctors Made in America* (Philadelphia: J. B. Lippincott, 1963); H. K. Skramstad, "The Engineer as Architect in Washington: The Contribution of Montgomery Meigs," in *Records of the Columbia Historical Society of Washington, D.C.,* edited by F. C. Rosenberger (Baltimore: Waverly Press, 1969–1970), pp. 266–284; A. Levinson, "The Three Meigs and Their Contribution to Pediatrics," *Annals of Medical History,* 1928, 10:138–148.

4. C. D. Meigs, *Obstetrics: The Science and the Art* (Philadelphia: Lea and Blanchard, 1849), pp. 364–376, 324; I. S. Cutter and H. R. Viets, *A Short History of Midwifery* (Philadelphia: W. B. Saunders, 1964); L. C. Scheffey, "The Earlier History and the Transition Period of Obstetrics and Gynecology in Philadelphia," *Annals of Medical History,* 1940, 2:215–224. Meigs was known for his strong opinions and his aggressive style. Being well respected as a physician did not mean that everyone agreed with everything he said. A comment that offends many people appeared in a medical

textbook, part of a long, rambling discourse on the role of women: "If we scan her position amidst the ornate circles of a Christian civilization, it is easy to perceive that her intellectual force is different from that of her master and lord. . . . The great administrative faculties are not hers. She plans no sublime campaigns, leads no armies to battle nor fleets to victory. The forum of no theater is for her silver voice, full of tenderness and sensibility. She discerns not the courses of the planets. . . . Home is her place, except when like the star of day, she deigns to issue forth to the world to exhibit her beauty and her grace and to scatter her smiles upon all that are worthy to receive so right a boon—then she goes back to her home, like as the sun sinks in the west. . . . She has a head almost too small for intellect and just big enough for love" (C. D. Meigs, *Females and Their Diseases* [Philadelphia: Lea and Blanchard, 1848], p. 40). Also see comments regarding public interest in Simpson's head size in Chapter 1.

5. R. W. Wertz and D. C. Wertz, *Lying-In: A History of Childbirth in America* (New York: Schocken Books, 1977), pp. 115–119; J. W. Leavitt, *Brought to Bed: Child-Bearing in America, 1750–1950* (New York: Oxford University Press, 1986), pp. 116–141; F. Palmer, *Priests of Lucinda: The Story of Obstetrics* (Boston: Little, Brown, 1939), pp. 222–244; I. Loudon, *Death in Childbirth: An International Study of Maternal Care and Maternal Mortality, 1800–1950* (New York: Oxford University Press, 1992), pp. 49–84.

6. W. Tyler-Smith, *Parturition and the Principles and Practice of Obstetrics* (Philadelphia: Blanchard and Lea, 1849), p. 177; P. Dubois, "On the Inhalation of Ether Applied to Cases of Midwifery," *Lancet*, 1847, 1:246; W. H. Byford, *A Treatise on the Theory and Practice of Obstetrics* (New York: William Wood, 1870), p. 23; F. H. Ramsbotham, *The Principles and Practice of Obstetric Medicine and Surgery in Reference to the Process of Parturition* (Philadelphia: Blanchard and Lea, 1855), p. 174; R. Collins, "Letter to C. D. Meigs, April 26, 1849," in *College of Physicians of Philadelphia*, Fugitive Leaves from the Library F1 152; Meigs, *Obstetrics*, pp. 364–376, 324.

7. E. Wagenknecht, *Mrs. Longfellow: Selected Letters and Journal of Fanny Appleton Longfellow* (New York: Longmans, Green, 1956), pp. 129–130; C. B. Pittinger, "The Anesthetization of Fanny

Longfellow for Childbirth on April 7, 1847," *Anesthesia and Analgesia*, 1987, 66:368–369; N. C. Keep, "The Letheon Administered in a Case of Labor," *Boston Medical and Surgical Journal*, 1847, 36:226; N. C. Keep, "Inhalation of Ethereal Vapor, or Mitigating Human Suffering in Surgical Operations and Acute Diseases," *Boston Medical and Surgical Journal*, 1847, 36:199–201; P. Keep, "Nathan Keep—William Morton's Salieri," *Anaesthesia*, 1995, 50: 233–238.

8. Wakley wrote: "Intense astonishment . . . has been excited through the profession by the rumour that her Majesty during her last labour was placed under the influence of chloroform, an agent which has unquestionably caused instantaneous death in a considerable number of cases. . . . We have felt irresistibly impelled to make the foregoing observations, fearing the consequences of allowing such a rumor respecting a dangerous practice in one of our national palaces to pass unrefuted. Royal examples are followed with extraordinary readiness by a certain class of society in this country" (*Lancet*, May 14, 1853, p. 453). The queen, after her anesthetic, is reputed to have said, "This blessed chloroform"—quoted in W. S. Sykes, "An Obstetric Scylla and Charybdis, or Victoria and Mr. Wakley," in Sykes, *Essays on the First Hundred Years of Anaesthesia* (Park Ridge, Ill.: Wood Library-Museum of Anesthesiology, 1982), pp. 77–85. C. Hibbert, *Queen Victoria in Her Letters and Journals—A Selection* (New York: Penguin Books, 1985), p. 97; D. Caton, "Obstetric Anesthesia: The First Ten Years," *Anesthesiology*, 1970, 33:102–109; J. S. Lewis, *In the Family Way: Childbearing in the British Aristocracy, 1760–1860* (New Brunswick, N.J.: Rutgers University Press, 1986), pp. 153–192.

9. M. S. Pernick, *A Calculus of Suffering: Pain, Professionalism, and Anesthesia in Nineteenth-Century America* (New York: Columbia University Press, 1985).

10. N. Pirogoff, *Researches Practical and Physiological on Etherization*, translated by B. R. Fink (Park Ridge, Ill.: Wood Library-Museum of Anesthesiology, 1992), pp. 3–4.

11. J. W. Comfort, *Thompsonian Practice of Midwifery and Treatment of Complaints Peculiar to Women and Children* (Philadelphia: Aaron Comfort, 1845), p. 39; T. Denman, *An Introduction*

to the Practice of Midwifery, 7th ed. (London: E. Cox, 1832), pp. 274–275; Meigs, *Obstetrics.*

12. Meigs, *Obstetrics;* Tyler-Smith, p. 177.

13. "Report of the Committee on Obstetrics," *Transactions of the American Medical Association,* 1848, 1:225–234; J. Snow, "On the Fatal Cases of Inhalation of Chloroform," *Edinburgh Medical Journal,* 1849, 72:75–87.

14. R. Barnes, "Further Observations on the Employment of Chloroform in Parturition," *Lancet,* 1848, 1:442–444.

15. Meigs, *Obstetrics;* Tyler-Smith; Ramsbotham; Barnes; F. W. Fischer, "Letter from Paris—Ethereal Inhalation in Insanity and Obstetrics," *Boston Medical and Surgical Journal,* 1847, 36:172–174; W. Osler, "Influence of Louis on American Medicine," *Bulletin of the Johns Hopkins Hospital,* August–September 1897, 8(77–78):161.

16. Ramsbotham; Barnes.

17. S. Ashwell, "Observations on the Use of Chloroform in Natural Labor," *Lancet,* 1848, 1:291–292.

18. W. Channing, *A Treatise on Etherization in Childbirth, Illustrated by Five Hundred Eighty-One Cases* (Boston: William Ticknor, 1848), p. 2; Snow; "Walter Channing, Obituary," *Boston Medical and Surgical Journal,* 1876, 95:237–238; H. Thoms, "Walter Channing and Etherization in Childbirth," *American Journal of Obstetrics and Gynecology,* 1930, 20:244; S. E. Morison, *Three Centuries of Harvard, 1636–1936* (Cambridge: Harvard University Press, 1936), p. 512.

19. Channing's dual appointment as professor of both medical jurisprudence and obstetrics may seem strange. At the time, however, neither discipline was thought important enough to warrant a separate chair—an interesting commentary on the status of obstetrics (*The Harvard Medical School, 1782–1906,* published in 1906 by the Medical School Faculty).

20. Channing, p. 2.

21. Channing's comments about ether's effects on labor were contradictory. In one paragraph he wrote that etherization could abolish contractions. He even recommended that it be used to control "the persistent contraction so common from ergotism" (p. 43). Yet he said that myometrial depression from etherization occurred

only in "exceptional cases" (p. 38). Later he wrote, "Etherization has no necessary effect to diminish the organic action of the womb" (p. 42), and, two pages after that: "Whatever ether's effect on the action of the uterus, it leads to a natural state of uterine function and consequently, [he] welcomes it" (p. 44). Caton, 1970; D. Caton, "Obstetric Anesthesia and Concepts of Placental Transport: A Historical Review of the Nineteenth Century," *Anesthesiology*, 1977, 46:132-137.

22. R. W. Johnstone, "William Cullen," *Medical History*, 1959, 3:33-46; J. B. Morrell, "The University of Edinburgh in the Late Eighteenth Century: Its Scientific Eminence and Academic Structure," *Isis*, 1971, 62:158-171; R. H. Shryock, "The Advent of Modern Medicine in Philadelphia, 1800-1850," *Yale Journal of Biology and Medicine*, 1941, 18:715-738; J. Z. Bowers, "The Influence of Edinburgh on American Medicine," in *Medical Education and Medical Care*, edited by G. McLachlan (Oxford: Oxford University Press, 1977), pp. 3-23; M. K. Kaufman, *American Medical Education: The Formative Years, 1765-1910* (London: Greenwood Press, 1976); L. C. Scheffey, "The Earlier History and the Transition Period of Obstetrics and Gynecology in Philadelphia," *Annals of Medical History*, 1940, 2:215-224.

Chapter Three
The Transformation of Medical Practice by Science

1. C. E. Rosenberg, "The Therapeutic Revolution: Medicine, Meaning, and Social Change in Nineteenth-Century America," in *The Therapeutic Revolution: Essays in the Social History of American Medicine*, edited by M. J. Vogel and C. E. Rosenberg (Philadelphia: University of Pennsylvania Press, 1979), pp. 3-26; M. P. Earles, "Experiments with Drugs and Poisons in the Seventeenth and Eighteenth Centuries," *Annals of Science*, 1963, 19:241-254; G. Kuschinsky, "The Influence of Dorpat on the Emergence of Pharmacology as a Distinct Discipline," *Journal of the History of Medicine*, 1968, 23:258-271; J. Koch-Weser and P. J. Schechter, "Smiedeberg in Strassburg, 1872-1918: The Making of Modern Pharmacology," *Life Sciences*, 1978, 22:1361-1372.

2. O. Temkin, *Galenism: Rise and Decline of a Medical Phi-

losophy (Ithaca: Cornell University Press, 1973); M. D. Grmerk, *Diseases in the Ancient Greek World,* translated by M. Muellner and L. Muellner (Baltimore: Johns Hopkins University Press, 1983); O. Temkin, *Hippocrates in a World of Pagans and Christians* (Baltimore: Johns Hopkins University Press, 1991); W. D. Smith, *The Hippocratic Tradition* (Ithaca: Cornell University Press, 1979).

3. L. S. King, *The Philosophy of Medicine: The Early Eighteenth Century* (Cambridge: Harvard University Press, 1978); G. B. Risse, "Medicine in the Age of Enlightenment," in *Medicine in Society,* edited by A. Wear (Cambridge: Cambridge University Press, 1992).

4. A. C. Chitnis, "Medical Education in Edinburgh, 1790-1826, and Some Victorian Social Consequences," *Medical History,* 1973, 17:178-185; R. W. Johnstone, "William Cullen," *Medical History,* 1959, 3:33-46.

5. G. B. Risse, "Doctor William Cullen, Physician, Edinburgh: A Consultation Practice in the Eighteenth Century," *Bulletin of the History of Medicine,* 1976, 48:338-351; *Medical Education and Medical Care, a Scottish-American Symposium,* edited by G. McLachlan (London: Oxford University Press for the Nuffield Provincial Hospitals Trust, 1977); C. Newman, *The Evolution of Medical Education in the Nineteenth Century* (New York: Oxford University Press, 1957); J. B. Morrell, "The University of Edinburgh in the Late Eighteenth Century: Its Scientific Eminence and Academic Structure," *Isis,* 1971, 62:158-171.

6. D. F. Hawke, *Benjamin Rush, Revolutionary Gadfly* (New York: Bobbs-Merrill, 1971); L. S. King, *Transformations in American Medicine: From Benjamin Rush to William Osler* (Baltimore: Johns Hopkins University Press, 1991); D. D. Runes, *The Selected Writings of Benjamin Rush* (New York: Philosophical Library, 1947).

7. J. Z. Bowers, *The Influence of Edinburgh on American Medicine in Medical Education and Medical Care* (London: Oxford University Press, 1977), pp. 2-23.

8. A. C. Siddall, "Bloodletting in American Obstetric Practice, 1800-1945," *Bulletin of the History of Medicine,* 1980, 54:101-110.

9. Siddall; M. P. Rucker, "An Eighteenth Century Method of Pain Relief in Obstetrics," *Journal of the History of Medicine and Allied Sciences,* 1950, 15:101-120.

10. G. B. Risse, "The Quest for Certainty in Medicine: John

Brown's System of Medicine in France," *Bulletin of the History of Medicine*, 1971, 45(1):1; C. A. Lopez, "Franklin and Mesmer: An Encounter," *Yale Journal of Biology and Medicine*, 1993, 66: 325–331; G. Rosen, "Mesmerism and Surgery: A Strange Chapter in the History of Anesthesia," *Journal of the History of Medicine*, 1946, 1:527–550; R. H. Shryock, *Medicine and Society in America, 1660–1860* (Ithaca: Cornell University Press, 1972), p. 127.

11. R. H. Shryock, "The Advent of Modern Medicine in Philadelphia, 1800–1850," *Yale Journal of Biology and Medicine*, 1941, 13:715–738.

12. R. H. Shryock, *The Development of Modern Medicine: An Interpretation of the Social and Scientific Factors Involved* (Madison: University of Wisconsin Press, 1979), pp. 72, 70; W. Corbett, quoted in *Medicine in America: Historical Essays* (Baltimore: Johns Hopkins University Press, 1966), p. 207; E. H. Ackerknecht, *Medicine at the Paris Hospital, 1794–1848* (Baltimore: Johns Hopkins University Press, 1967), pp. 102–104.

13. R. C. Maulitz, "Channel Crossing: The Lure of French Pathology for English Medical Students, 1816–36," *Bulletin of the History of Medicine*, 1981, 55:475–496.

14. Ackerknecht; W. Osler, "Influence of Louis on American Medicine," *Bulletin of the Johns Hopkins Hospital*, August–September 1897, 8(77–78):161.

15. K. Thomas, *Man and the Natural World: A History of Modern Sensibility* (New York: Pantheon Books, 1983), pp. 92–191; J. Turner, *Reckoning with the Beast: Animals, Pain and Humanity in the Victorian Mind* (Baltimore: Johns Hopkins University Press, 1980).

16. J. H. Cassedy, *American Medicine and Statistical Thinking, 1800–1860* (Cambridge: Harvard University Press, 1984).

17. J. E. Lesch, *Science and Medicine in France: The Emergence of Experimental Physiology, 1790–1855* (Cambridge: Harvard University Press, 1984).

18. Shryock, *Medicine and Society in America*, p. 127; R. V. Bruce, *The Launching of Modern American Science, 1846–1876* (Ithaca: Cornell University Press, 1987); L. C. Scheffey, "The Earlier History and the Transition Period of Obstetrics and Gynecology in Philadelphia," *Annals of Medical History*, May 1940, 2:215–224;

Standing Committee on Medical Literature, "Original Medical Publications by American Authors: Committee Report," *Transactions of the American Medical Association*, 1851, 4:482.

19. S. Bard, *A Compendium on the Theory and Practice of Midwifery Containing Practical Instructions for the Management of Women During Pregnancy, in Labour and in Child-Bed* (New York: Collins, 1812), p. 91.

20. W. Leishman, *A System of Midwifery* (Glasgow: James Maclehose, 1873), p. 242; C. D. Meigs, *Obstetrics: The Science and the Art* (Philadelphia: Lea and Blanchard, 1849), p. 401; J. Y. Simpson, "Lecture Notes on Eclampsia," in *Selected Obstetrical and Gynaecological Works*, edited by J. W. Black (Edinburgh: Adam and Charles Black, 1871), pp. 57-59.

21. M. P. Rucker, "An Eighteenth Century Method of Pain Relief in Obstetrics," *Journal of the History of Medicine and Allied Sciences*, 1950, 15:101-120; J. Y. Simpson, "On the Inhalation of Sulphuric Ether in the Practice of Midwifery," *Edinburgh Monthly Journal of Medical Science*, March 1847, pp. 721-732.

22. Standing Committee on Medical Literature.

23. W. Channing, *A Treatise on Etherization in Childbirth, Illustrated by Five Hundred Eighty-One Cases* (Boston: William Ticknor, 1848); G. H. Daniels, *American Science in the Age of Jackson* (New York: Columbia University Press, 1968); C. Bernard, *Introduction to the Study of Experimental Medicine*, translated by H. C. Greene and L. J. Henderson (New York: Macmillan, 1927), pp. 129-150. Claude Bernard believed that "the application of mathematics to natural phenomena is the aim of all science." However, he also thought it necessary to first identify all the physiologic variables through "comparative experimentation." He did not disagree with the use of mathematics and statistics in principle, only in practice.

Chapter Four
John Snow's Approach to Anesthesia

1. *The Case Books of Dr. John Snow* (London: Wellcome Institute for the History of Medicine, 1994), pp. ix-x, 47; D. A. E. Shephard, *John Snow: Anaesthetist to a Queen and Epidemiolo-*

gist to a Nation (Cornwall: York Point Publishing, 1995); B. W. Richardson, "The Life of John Snow," in *On Chloroform and Other Anaesthetics,* by John Snow (London: John Churchill, 1858), pp. l–lxiv, 79, 325. Virtually all available information about Snow comes from this short biography, a foreword to Snow's book, which was published posthumously. Benjamin Ward Richardson, a physician, was a close friend of Snow's and was probably still recovering from the loss when he wrote the biography.

2. J. Snow, *On the Inhalation of the Vapour of Ether in Surgical Operations* (London: John Churchill, 1847), pp. 1, 13; Richardson; *Case Books of Dr. John Snow,* 847, pp. ix–x; Shephard.

3. J. Snow, "On Asphyxia, and on the Resuscitation of Stillborn Children," *London Medical Gazette,* 1841–1842, 1:222–227.

4. Considerable detail about Snow's studies of cholera may be found in Shephard's biography of John Snow.

5. Snow, *On the Inhalation of the Vapour.*

6. E. H. Ackerknecht, "Aspects of the History of Therapeutics," *Bulletin of the History of Medicine,* 1962, 36:389–418; M. P. Earles, "Experiments with Drugs and Poisons in the Seventeenth and Eighteenth Centuries," *Annals of Science,* 1965, 19:241–254; J. Kock-Weser and P. J. Schechter, "Schmiedeberg in Strassburg, 1872–1918: The Making of Modern Pharmacology," *Life Sciences,* 1978, 22:1361–1372; G. Kuschinsky, "The Influence of Dorpat on the Emergence of Pharmacology as a Distinct Discipline," *Journal of the History of Medicine,* 1968, 23:258–271.

7. Richardson, pp. l–lxiv, 79, 325; Snow, Flourens, and Bernard described the clinical signs of anesthesia.

8. Several early investigators speculated about the mechanism of anesthesia, among them Claude Bernard in *Lectures on Anesthetics and on Asphyxia,* translated by B. R. Fink (Park Ridge, Ill.: Wood Library-Museum of Anesthesiology, 1989), and Nicholas Pirogoff, a Russian surgeon, in *Recherches pratiques et physiologiques sur l'éthérisation,* translated by B. R. Fink (Park Ridge, Ill.: Wood Library-Museum of Anesthesiology, 1992).

9. Richardson.

10. J. Snow, "On the Administration of Chloroform During Parturition," *Association of Medicine Journal,* 1853, 1:500–502.

11. H. Thoms, "Anesthesia à la Reine—A Chapter in the History

of Anesthesia," *American Journal of Obstetrics and Gynecology*, 1940, 40:340-346.

12. Richardson.

13. J. Snow, "On the Fatal Cases of Inhalation of Chloroform," *Edinburgh Medical and Surgical Journal*, 1849, 72:75-87.

14. S. C. Thommson, "The Great Windmill Street School," *Bulletin of the History of Medicine*, 1942, 12:377-391; D. van Zwanenberg, "The Training and Careers of Those Apprenticed to Apothecaries in Suffolk, 1815-1858," *Medical History*, 1983, 27: 139-150; F. N. L. Poynter, "Medical Education in England Since 1600," in *The History of Medical Education*, edited by C. D. O'Malley (Los Angeles: University of California Press, 1970), pp. 235-250.

15. Although the medical curriculum of the Hunterian School did include chemistry, clinicians, not scientists, taught the subject. We do not know if their lectures included the physics or chemistry of gases, but it seems unlikely. Medical schools in England emphasized applied medicine, not science. Nor is it likely that Snow learned about the physics of gases while attending meetings of the Westminster Medical Society. We know of the lectures given at this society through announcements and lecture notes published in the *Lancet*, 1839-1840, 1:222-231 and 1:307-317. None of those listed were pertinent to Snow's work, with the exception of a series of lectures by the London surgeon Henry Ancell. Two of his lectures deal with the composition of blood, but in neither does he discuss problems of solubility, absorption, or transport, the areas that Snow explored. Thommson; van Zwanenberg; Poynter; T. Gelfand, "Invite the Philosopher, as Well as the Charitable: Hospital Teaching as Private Enterprise in Hunterian London," in *William Hunter and the Eighteenth-Century Medical World*, edited by W. F. Bynum and R. Porter (Cambridge: Cambridge University Press, 1985), pp. 7-34.

16. N. A. Bergman, "Michael Faraday and His Contribution to Anesthesia," *Anesthesiology*, 1992, 77:812-816; N. A. Bergman, "Forerunners of Modern Anesthesiology: Dwarfs and Giants," *Pharos*, Fall 1985, pp. 8-12; F. F. Cartwright, "Humphry Davy's Contribution to Anaesthesia," *Proceedings of the Royal Society of Medicine*, 1950, 42:571-578; Richardson.

17. Other physicians commented on Simpson's ability to attract public attention. One physician who had been embroiled in a controversy with Simpson wrote, "We shall see . . . whether Dr. Simpson himself does not flee off to some new marvel, some fresher novelty, to attract public notoriety, and to cover his defeat in the BATTLE OF PLACENTA PRAEVIA!" The statement was prophetic, because Simpson did just that. The same issue of the *Lancet* contains Simpson's paper describing his first use of chloroform (*Lancet,* 1847, p. 549).

18. W. Tyler-Smith, *A Course of Lectures on Obstetrics* (New York: Robert M. DeWill, 1858), p. 732; F. H. Ramsbotham, *The Principles and Practice of Obstetric Medicine and Surgery,* 5th ed. (London: John Churchill and Sons, 1867), p. 197.

19. Simpson's critics remained cautious and critical, however. Commenting on the changing mood in Paris, Fischer observed that the "enthusiasm which had hitherto prevailed in regard to ether, has gradually subsided, and the subject is now becoming one of cool and scientific consideration" (F. W. Fischer, "Letter from Paris—Ethereal Inhalation," *Boston Medical and Surgical Journal,* March 1, 1847, 36:172-174).

Chapter Five
Balancing the Risks of Pain and Anesthesia

1. W. J. Little, "On the Influence of Abnormal Parturition, Difficult Labors, Premature Birth, and Asphyxia Neonatorum, on the Mental and Physical Condition of the Child, Especially in Relation to Deformities," *Transactions of the Obstetrical Society of London,* 1861, pp. 293-344.

2. D. Caton, "Obstetric Anesthesia: The First Ten Years," *Anesthesiology,* 1970, 33:102-109; J. Snow, "On Administration of Chloroform During Parturition," *Association of Medicine Journal,* 1853, 1:500-502.

3. F. H. Ramsbotham, *The Principles and Practice of Obstetric Medicine and Surgery in Reference to the Process of Parturition* (Philadelphia: Blanchard and Lea, 1855), p. 177.

4. W. Channing, *A Treatise on Etherization in Childbirth,*

Illustrated by Five Hundred Eighty-One Cases (Boston: William Ticknor, 1848).

5. Aristotle, *Generation of Animals*, translated by A. L. Peck (Cambridge: Harvard University Press, 1943), pp. 197-201; W. Harvey, *Anatomical Exercises on the Generation of Animals: The Works of W. Harvey, M.D.*, translated by R. Willis (London: Sydenham Society, 1858), p. 473; W. J. Mayow, "Tractatus Quinque Medico-Physici," quoted in *Chemical Embryology*, by J. Needham (New York: Hafner, 1963), p. 173; W. B. Carpenter, *Principles of Human Physiology and Comparative Anatomy* (Philadelphia: Blanchard and Lea, 1858), pp. 133-135, 769-771.

6. Carpenter; S. Schauenstein, "Über den Übergang Medikamentöser Stoffe aus der Kreislaufe der Saugenden, in ihre Milch und aus dem Kreislaufe der Schwangeren in ihr Fruchtwasser und ihren Fötus," *Jahrbuch für Kinderheilkunde und Physische Erziehung*, 1858-1859, 2:13-18; J. Pereira, *The Elements of Materia Medica and Therapeutics*, 2d ed. (London: Longman, Brown and Green, 1842); A. Harvey, "On the Foetus in Utero, as Inoculating the Maternal with the Peculiarities of the Paternal Organism; and on Mental States in Either Parent, as Influencing Nutrition and Development of the Offspring," *Edinburgh Journal of Medical Science*, 1849, pp. 1130-1143; 1850, pp. 299-310; 1850, pp. 387-398.

7. Caton.

8. D. I. Macht, "The History of Opium and Some of Its Preparations and Alkaloids," *Journal of American Medical Association*, 1915, 64:477-481; H. H. Kane, *The Hypodermic Injection of Morphia: Its History, Advantages and Dangers* (New York: Charles L. Bermingham, 1880); E. Kormann, "Die Anwendung subcutaner Morphium-Injection unter der Geburt und in den ersten Tagedes Wochenbettes," *Monatsschrift für Geburtskunde und Frauenkrankheiten*, 1868, 32:114-127; Schauenstein.

9. F. Ramsbotham, "Lectures on the Theory and Practice of Midwifery," *London Medical Gazette*, 1834, 14:81-87; Pereira.

10. C. E. Terry and M. E. Perkins, *The Opium Problem* (Committee on Drug Addiction, in Collaboration with the Bureau of Social Hygiene, 1928), pp. 410-426.

11. J. J. Lamadrid, "A Case Illustrating the Influence on the

Infant of Medicines, Particularly Narcotics, Administered to the Mother During Pregnancy and Labor," *American Journal of Obstetrics and Gynecology,* 1877, 10:466–469; "Chloral and the Foetus in Utero," *American Journal of Obstetrics and Gynecology,* 1871–1872, 4:759–760; "Mittheilungen aus der Gesellschaft für Geburtshilfe in Leipzig," *Archiv für Gynaekologie,* 1876, 10:188–189; "The Influence on the Foetus of Medicines, Particularly Narcotics, Administered to the Mother During Pregnancy and Labor, Transactions of the New York Obstetrical Society (Meeting February 6, 1877)," *American Journal of Obstetrics and Gynecology,* 1877, 10: 300–335.

12. Caton; W. Reitz, "Über die passiven Wanderungen der Zinnoberkörnchen durch den thierischen Organismus," *Centralblatt für die Medizinischen Wissenschaften,* 1868, 41:654–655; F. A. Hoffmann and P. Langerhans, "Über den Verbleib des in die Circulation eingeführten Zinnobers," *Archiv der Pathölogischen Anatomie,* 1863, 48:303–325; W. S. Savory, "An Experimental Inquiry into the Effect upon the Mother of Poisoning the Foetus," *Lancet,* 1858, 1:362–364, 385–386.

13. C. C. Hüter, "Beobachtung über die Wirkungen des Chloroforms bei Geburtshilflichen Operationen," *Neue Zeitschrift für Geburtskunde,* 1850, 27:321–391; A. Döderlein, "Zum Gedächtnis P. Zweifel," *Archiv für Gynaekologie,* 1927, 131:i–viii.

14. P. Zweifel, "Einfluss der Chloroformnarcose Kreissender auf den Fötus," *Berliner Klinische Wochenschrift,* 1874, 11:245–247; P. Zweifel, "Der Übergang von Chloroform und Salizylsäure in die Placenta, nebst Bemerkungen über den Icterus Neonatorum," *Archiv für Gynaekologie,* 1877, 12:235–257.

15. R. H. Shryock, *Medicine and Society in America* (Ithaca: Cornell University Press, 1972).

16. Döderlein; W. Nagel, "Adolf Gusserow," *Deutsche Medizine Wochenschrift,* 1906, 32:430; H. Thierfelder, *Felix Hoppe-Seyler* (Enke, 1926).

17. A. Gusserow, "Zur Lehre vom Stoffwechsel des Foetus," *Archiv für Gynaekologie,* 1871, 3:241–270; A. Gusserow, "Zur Lehre vom Stoffaustausch zwischen Mutter und Frucht," *Archiv für Gynaekologie,* 1878, 13:56–72.

18. Gusserow, "Zur Lehre vom Stoffwechsel des Foetus."

19. Gusserow, "Zur Lehre vom Stoffwechsel des Foetus."

20. P. Zweifel, "Die Respiration des Fötus," *Archiv für Gynae-kologie,* 1876, 9:291-305.

21. H. Fehling, "Zur Lehre vom Stoffwechsel zwischen Mutter und Frucht," *Archiv für Gynaekologie,* 1876, 9:313-318; Benecke, "Zur Lehre vom Stoffwechsel zwischen Mutter und Frucht," *Archiv für Gynaekologie,* 1875, 8:536-537; H. Fehling, "Beiträge zur Physiologie des Placentaren Stoffverkehrs," *Archiv für Gynaekologie,* 1877, 11:523-557.

22. F. W. Scanzoni, "Über die Anwendung der Anaesthetica in der geburtshilflichen Praxis," *Beiträge zur Geburtskunde und Gynaekologie,* 1855, 2:62-93; C. Kidd, "On the Value of Anaesthetic Aid in Midwifery," *Transactions of Obstetrical Society of London,* 1860, 2:340-361; A. E. Sansom, "On the Pain of Parturition and Anaesthetics in Obstetric Practice," *Transactions of Obstetrical Society of London,* 1868, 10:121-140.

Chapter Six
The Social Connotations of Pain

1. M. S. Pernick, *A Calculus of Suffering: Pain, Professionalism and Anesthesia in Nineteenth Century America* (New York: Columbia University Press, 1985).

2. R. H. Ellis, "The Introduction of Ether Anaesthesia to Great Britain," *Anaesthesia,* 1976, 31:766-777; W. S. Sykes, *Essays on the First Hundred Years of Anaesthesia,* vol. 1 (New York: Churchill Livingstone, 1982), pp. 48-76, 117-136; W. K. Frankel, "The Introduction of General Anesthesia in Germany," *Journal of the History of Medicine,* 1946, 1:612-617; E. H. Hume, "Peter Parker and the Introduction of Anesthesia into China," *Journal of the History of Medicine,* 1946, 1:670-674; D. I. Macht, "History of Opium and Some of the Preparations and Alkaloids," *Journal of the American Medical Association,* 1915, 64:477-481; B. R. Fink, "Leaves and Needles: The Introduction of Surgical Local Anesthesia," *Anesthesiology,* 1985, 63:77-83; T. E. Keys, *The History of Surgical Anesthesia* (New York: Dover, 1963); J. C. Trent, "Surgical Anesthesia, 1846-1946," *Journal of the History of Medicine,* 1946, 1:505-514; W. D. A. Smith, *Under the Influence: A History*

of Nitrous Oxide and Oxygen Anaesthesia (Park Ridge, Ill.: Wood Library-Museum of Anesthesiology, 1982), pp. 30, 2; F. L. Taylor, "Crawford Williamson Long," *Annals of Medical History,* 1945, 7: 267-296; F. K. Boland, *The First Anesthetic: The Story of Crawford Long* (Athens: University of Georgia Press, 1950); D. Caton, "The Secularization of Pain," *Anesthesiology,* 1985, 62:493-501.

3. W. James, *The Varieties of Religious Experience: A Study in Human Nature* (New York: Penguin Books, 1982), pp. 297-298.

4. O. Chadwick, *The Secularization of the European Mind in the Nineteenth Century* (New York: Cambridge University Press, 1977).

5. J. J. Pollitt, *Art and Experience in Classical Greece* (New York: Cambridge University Press, 1972), pp. 30-31; E. Schillebeeckx, *Christ: The Experience of Jesus as Lord,* translated by J. Bowden (New York: Crossroad, 1981), p. 671; C. S. Lewis, *The Problem of Pain* (New York: Macmillan, 1962), p. 16.

6. E. Pagel, *Adam, Eve, and the Serpent* (New York: Random· House, 1988), pp. 98-150; M. D. Grmek, *Diseases in the Ancient Greek World,* translated by M. Muellner and L. Muellner (Baltimore: Johns Hopkins University Press, 1989).

7. Homer, *The Odyssey,* translated by R. Fitzgerald (New York: Doubleday, 1963), p. 2; Aeschylus, *The Oresteia,* translated by R. Fagles (New York: Penguin Books, 1984), p. 243.

8. Pagel; O. Temkin, "Medicine and the Problem of Moral Responsibility," *Bulletin of the History of Medicine,* 1949, 23:1-20.

9. G. Boccaccio, *The Decameron,* edited by R. Allison (New York: Basic Books, 1982), pp. 39-42; C. S. Bartsocas, "Two Fourteenth-Century Greek Descriptions of the 'Black Death,'" *Journal of the History of Medicine,* 1966, 21:394-400; N. Cohn, *The Pursuit of the Millennium* (New York: Oxford University Press, 1970); P. Ziegler, *The Black Death* (New York: Harper and Row, 1969); K. Thomas, *Religion and the Decline of Magic* (New York: Charles Scribner's Sons, 1971), p. 77; C. M. Cipolla, *Faith, Reason, and the Plague in Seventeenth-Century Tuscany* (New York: W. W. Norton, 1981); S. R. Ell, "Concepts of Disease and the Physician in the Early Middle Ages," *Janus,* 1978, 65:153-175.

10. J. Pelikan, *Jesus Through the Centuries* (New Haven: Yale University Press, 1985), pp. 95-108.

11. J. Huizinga, *The Waning of the Middle Ages* (New York: Doubleday, 1954); J. H. Langbein, *Torture and the Law of Proof: Europe and England in the Ancient Régime* (Chicago: University of Chicago Press, 1977); P. Spierenburg, *The Spectacle of Suffering: Executions and the Evolution of Repression from Preindustrial Metropolis to the European Experience* (New York: Cambridge University Press, 1984); P. Brown, *Society and the Holy in Late Antiquity* (Berkeley: University of California Press, 1982), p. 131; Thomas; *The Song of Roland,* translated by G. Burgess (London: Penguin Books, 1990), p. 77.

12. G. G. Dawson, *Healing: Pagan and Christian* (New York: AMS Press, 1977), p. 152; Grmek; Ell; W. D. Smith, *The Hippocratic Tradition* (Ithaca: Cornell University Press, 1979); D. W. Amundsen, "Medicine and Faith in Early Christianity," *Bulletin of the History of Medicine,* 1982, 56:326-350; J. Kroll and B. Bachrach, "Sin and the Etiology of Disease in Pre-Crusade Europe," *Journal of the History of Medicine and Allied Science,* 1986, 41:395-414; B. Farrington, *Greek Science* (Baltimore: Penguin Books, 1966), pp. 66-78; O. Tempkin, *Hippocrates in a World of Pagans and Christians* (Baltimore: Johns Hopkins University Press, 1991), pp. 94-105.

13. R. H. Shryock, *Medicine in America: Historical Essays* (Baltimore: Johns Hopkins University Press, 1966); R. S. Gottfried, *The Black Death: Natural and Human Disaster in Medieval Europe* (New York: Free Press, 1983); P. Starr, *The Social Transformation of American Medicine* (New York: Basic Books, 1982), pp. 39-40; A. E. Clark-Kennedy, *Stephen Hales, an Eighteenth Century Biography* (Cambridge: Cambridge University Press, 1929).

14. C. Mather, *The Angel of Bethesda: An Essay upon the Common Maladies of Mankind,* edited by G. W. Jones (Barre: American Antiquarian Society of Barre, 1972), pp. 233-248; O. T. Beall, Jr., and R. H. Shryock, *Cotton Mather: First Significant Figure in American Medicine* (Baltimore: Johns Hopkins University Press, 1954); J. Wesley, *Primitive Remedies* (Santa Barbara: Woodbridge Press, 1975), pp. 9-11.

15. Wesley; Mather.

16. Mather.

17. Soranus, *Gynecology,* edited by O. Temkin, N. J. Eastman,

L. Edelstein, and A. F. Guttmacher (Baltimore: Johns Hopkins University Press, 1991), p. 72.

18. J. Donne, "An Anatomy of the World," in *The Complete English Poems,* edited by A. J. Smith (New York: Penguin Books, 1981), p. 273; F. N. L. Poynter, "John Donne and William Harvey," *Journal of the History of Medicine,* 1960, 15:233-246.

19. I. Loudon, *Death in Childbirth: An International Study of Maternal Care and Maternal Mortality, 1800-1950* (Oxford: Clarendon Press, 1992); A. Bradstreet, "Before the Birth of One of Her Children," in *The Complete Works of Anne Bradstreet,* edited by J. R. McGrath and A. P. Robb (Boston: Twayne, 1981), pp. 21-23.

20. *The Book of Common Prayer* (New York: Henry Holt, 1992), p. 320; T. R. Forbes, "The Regulation of English Midwives in the Sixteenth and Seventeenth Centuries," *Medical History,* 1964, 7:235-243; R. L. Petrelli, "The Regulation of French Midwifery During the *Ancien Régime,*" *Journal of the History of Medicine,* 1971, 26:276-292.

21. J. Y. Simpson, "Answers to the Religious Objections Advanced Against the Employment of Anaesthetic Agents in Surgery and Obstetrics in Anaesthesia, Hospitalism, Hermaphrodites and a Proposal to Stamp Out Small-Pox and Other Contagious Diseases," in *The Collected Works of James Young Simpson,* vol. 2, edited by W. G. Simpson (Edinburgh: Adam and Charles Black, 1874), pp. 42-64; P. Smith, "Scriptural Authority for the Mitigation of the Pains of Labour by Chloroform and Other Anaesthetic Agents," and J. Y. Simpson, Letter to Protheroe Smith, both also in *Simpson's Collected Works,* vol. 2.

22. S. Ashwell, "Observations on the Use of Chloroform in Natural Labour," *Lancet,* 1848, 1:481-482.

23. Dawson; A. D. Farr, "Religious Opposition to Obstetric Anaesthesia: A Myth?" *Annals of Science,* 1983, 40:159-177; J. Duns, *Memoir of Sir James Y. Simpson* (Edinburgh: Bart, Edmonston and Douglas, 1873).

Chapter Seven
Pain as Biological and Anesthesia as Necessary

1. J. Y. Simpson, "On the Inhalation of Sulphuric Ether in the Practice of Midwifery," *Edinburgh Monthly Journal of Medical Science*, March 1847, pp. 721–732.

2. W. Blake, "On Another's Sorrow," in *The Complete Poetry and Prose of William Blake*, edited by D. V. Erdman (New York: Doubleday, Anchor, 1982), p. 17.

3. W. Blake, "Visions of the Daughters of Albion," in *The Complete Poetry and Prose of William Blake*, edited by D. V. Erdman (New York: Doubleday, Anchor, 1982), p. 49; W. Wordsworth, "Ode on Intimations of Immortality from Recollections of Early Childhood," in *The Literature of England*, 3d ed., edited by G. B. Woods, H. A. Watt, and G. K. Anderson (Chicago: Scott, Foresman, 1953), p. 681; G. Himmelfarb, *The Idea of Poverty: England in the Early Industrial Age* (New York: Knopf, 1984).

4. W. D. A. Smith, *Under the Influence: A History of Nitrous Oxide and Oxygen Anaesthesia* (Park Ridge, Ill.: Wood Library-Museum of Anesthesiology, 1982), pp. 30, 2.

5. J. Locke, *An Essay Concerning Human Understanding* (London: Everyman's Library, 1947), pp. 16, 55.

6. J. Bentham, *Introduction to the Principles of Morals and Legislation*, edited by J. H. Burons and H. L. A. Hart (New York: Methuen, 1982), p. 34.

7. J. S. Mill, *Nature and Utilitarianism*, edited by M. Cohen (New York: Modern Library, 1961), pp. 463-467, 330.

8. P. Gay, *The Enlightenment: An Interpretation—The Rise of Modern Paganism* (New York: W. W. Norton, 1977), p. 6.

9. S. Hales, *Statical Essays; Containing Haemastaticks* (New York: Hafner, 1964), pp. xix-xx.

10. F. Bacon, "Of Fortune," in *Selected Writings*, edited by H. G. Dick (New York: Random House, 1955), p. 105; L. S. King, *The Philosophy of Medicine: The Early Eighteenth Century* (Cambridge: Harvard University Press, 1978); C. C. Booth, "Clinical Science in the Age of Reason," *Perspectives in Biology and Medicine*, 1981, 25:932-114.

11. H. Merskey, "Some Features of the History of the Idea of

Pain," *Pain*, 1980, 9:3–8. Comparisons of pain are difficult because no objective criteria exist for measuring, much less comparing, the pain of individuals or of groups. Investigators work around this problem by subjecting volunteers to pain stimuli of known intensity—a measured amount of electrical current or heat, for example. The subject is then asked to rate the pain on a relative scale, from trivial to the worst imaginable. To compare the intensity of pain within a culture at different times in history is, of course, impossible. Regardless, contemporary physiologists believe that the physical experience of pain has not changed. We can only speculate whether renal colic or childbirth produces more pain now than it did a millennium ago. Comparing estimates of pain among contemporary groups, physiologists believe that culture and education do not affect the physical (as opposed to perceived) intensity of physical pain. They do acknowledge that cultural and social patterns may influence the response of an individual to a pain of given intensity. Some cultures value stoicism more than others. See D. DeMoulin, "A Historical-Phenomenological Study of Bodily Pain in Western Man," *Bulletin of the History of Medicine*, 1974, 48:540–570; R. Melsack, "The Myth of Painless Childbirth," *Pain*, 1984, 19:321–337.

12. T. M. Brown, "From Mechanism to Vitalism in Eighteenth-Century English Physiology," *Journal of the History of Biology*, 1974, 7:179–216; K. M. Figlio, "Theories of Perception and the Physiology of Mind in the Late Eighteenth Century," *History of Science*, 1975, 12:177–212.

13. R. Whytt, *Observation on the Nature, Causes, and Cure of Those Disorders Which Have Been Commonly Called Nervous, Hypochondriac or Hysteric*, 2d ed. (Edinburgh: J Balfour, 1765), pp. 4, v–vii.

14. Whytt.

15. C. Lawrence, "The Nervous System and Society in the Scottish Enlightenment," in *Natural Order in Historical Studies of Scientific Culture*, edited by B. Barnes and S. Shapin (London: Sage Publications, 1979), pp. 19–40.

16. Lawrence; King.

17. C. Sherrington, *The Integrative Action of the Nervous System* (New Haven: Yale University Press, 1961).

18. L. C. McHenry, *Garrison's History of Neurology* (Springfield, Ill.: Thomas, 1969); K. M. Dallenbach, "Pain: History and Present Status," *American Journal of Psychology*, 1939, 52:331–347; H. K. Beecher, "The Measurement of Pain," *Pharmacological Reviews*, 1957, 9:59–209.

19. J. S. Jewell, "Influence of Our Present Civilization in the Production of Nervous and Mental Diseases," *Journal of Nervous and Mental Diseases*, 1881, 8(1):1–24; S. W. Mitchell, "Civilization and Pain," *Journal of the American Medical Association*, 1892, 18: 108.

20. T. Denman, *An Introduction to the Practice of Midwifery* (Brattleborough: W. Fessenden, 1807), pp. 187–190; G. J. Engelmann, *Labor Among Primitive Peoples: Showing the Development of the Obstetric Science of Today from the Natural and Instinctive Customs of All Races, Civilized and Savage, Past and Present* (Saint Louis: J. H. Chambers, 1882), p. 130; E. C. Stanton, "Letter to Susan B. Anthony, April 2, 1852," quoted in *The Oven Birds: American Women on Womanhood, 1830–1920*, edited by Gail Parker (Garden City, N.Y.: Doubleday Books, 1972), p. 260.

21. G. D. Read, *Revelation of Childbirth* (London: Heinemann, 1943).

22. R. H. Gabriel, *The Course of American Democratic Thought*, 2d ed. (New York: Ronald Press, 1956).

23. C. J. Sommerville, *The Rise and Fall of Childhood* (Beverly Hills, Calif.: Sage Publications, 1982); J. Walvin, *A Child's World: A Social History of English Childhood, 1800–1914* (New York: Penguin Books, 1982); J. Schiller, "Claude Bernard and Vivisection," *Journal of the History of Medicine*, 1967, 45:246–260; L. G. Stevenson, "Religious Elements in the Background of the British Anti-Vivisection Movement," *Yale Journal of Biology and Medicine*, 1956, 29:125–157; A. N. Rowan and B. E. Rollins, "Animal Research For and Against: A Philosophical, Social, and Historical Perspective," *Perspectives in Biology and Medicine*, 1983, 27:1–17; J. Turner, *Reckoning with the Beast* (Baltimore: Johns Hopkins University Press, 1980).

24. "Letter from J. Y. Simpson to Mr. Waldie of Liverpool, 14 November 1847," in *Simpson's Collected Works*, vol. 2, ed. W. G. Simpson (Edinburgh: Adam and Charles Black, 1874).

25. R. Nisbet, *History of the Idea of Progress* (New York: Basic Books, 1970); J. S. Mill, "Utilitarianism," in *The Six Great Essays of John Stuart Mill,* edited by A. W. Levi (New York: Washington Square Press, 1963), p. 257; E. H. Clarke, "Practical Medicine," in *A Century of American Medicine, 1776-1876* (Brinklow: Old Hickory Bookshop, 1963), pp. 6-13; O. W. Holmes, quoted in *Anesthetics in Labor,* by S. S. Todd, reprinted from the *Transactions of the American Medical Association of the State of Missouri for 1875,* p. 25.

26. *Queen Victoria in Her Letters and Journals,* edited by C. Hibbert (Great Britain: Penguin Books, 1985), p. 97; *Letters of Queen Victoria from the Archives of the House of Brandenburg-Prussia,* translated by Mrs. J. Pudney and Lord Sudley and edited by H. Bolitho (New Haven: Yale University Press, 1938), p. 104.

27. J. Duffy, "Anglo-American Reaction to Obstetrical Anesthesia," *Bulletin of the History of Medicine,* 1964, 38:32-44; S. D. Hoffert, *Private Matters: American Attitudes Toward Childbearing and Infant Nurture in the Urban North, 1800-1860* (Urbana: University of Illinois Press, 1989), pp. 89-91.

28. W. T. Smith, *A Course of Lectures on Obstetrics,* 2d ed. (New York: R. M. DeWitt, 1858), pp. 732-752; W. T. Lusk, *The Science and Art of Midwifery* (New York: D. Appleton, 1889), p. 227; W. H. Byford, *A Treatise on the Theory and Practice of Obstetrics* (New York: William Wood, 1870), p. 22; G. Marx and T. Katsnelson, "The Introduction of Nitrous Analgesia into Obstetrics," *Obstetrics and Gynecology,* 1992, 80:715-718; S. S. Todd, "Anesthetics in Labor," reprinted from the *Transactions of the Medical Association of the State of Missouri for 1875,* pp. 1-21.

29. *Report of the Committee Appointed by the Royal Medical and Surgical Society to Enquire into the Uses and the Physiological, Therapeutic and Toxical Effects of Chloroform* (London: J. E. Adlard, 1864); A. W. H. Lea, *Puerperal Infection* (London: H. Froude, 1910), p. 27; Mitchell, p. 108.

30. M. Murrey, "Presidential Address to the Obstetrical Society of Edinburgh, 1906," quoted in *Oliver Wendell Holmes and Puerperal Fever,* by C. J. Collingsworth (London: H. J. Glaisher, 1906); W. A. N. Dorland, *A Manual of Obstetrics* (Philadelphia: W. B. Saunders, 1896), p. 172.

Chapter Eight
The American Women's Campaign for Twilight Sleep

1. R. H. Shryock, *The Development of Modern Medicine: An Interpretation of the Social and Scientific Factors Involved* (Madison: University of Wisconsin Press, 1974), pp. 116–119.

2. R. von Steinbüchel, "Voläufige Mittheilung über die Anwendung von Skopolamin-Morphium-Injectionen in der Geburtshilfe," *Zentralblatt für Gynaekologie,* 1902, 30:1304–1306; C. J. Gauss, "Die Anwendung des Skopolamin-Morphium Dämmerschlafes in der Geburtshilfe," *Medizinische Klinik,* 1906, 2:136–138.

3. C. Lawrence, "Experiment and Experience in Anaesthesia: Alfred Goodman Levy and Chloroform Death, 1910–1960," in *Medical Theory, Surgical Practice: Studies in the History of Surgery,* edited by C. Lawrence (London: Routledge, 1992), pp. 263–294; B. M. Duncum, *The Development of Inhalation Anesthesia* (London: Royal Society of Medicine Press, 1994), pp. 426–456.

4. M. Tracy and C. Leupp, "Painless Childbirth," *McClure's Magazine,* June 1914, 413:37–51.

5. V. G. Drachman, *Hospital with a Heart: Women, Doctors, and the Paradox of Separatism at the New England Hospital, 1862–1969* (Ithaca: Cornell University Press, 1984); M. N. Kleinert, "Medical Women in New England: History of the New England Women's Medical Society," *Journal of American Medical Women's Association,* 1956, 2:63–67; V. A. Metaxas Quiroga, "Female Lay Managers and Scientific Pediatrics at Nursery and Child's Hospital, 1854–1910," *Bulletin of the History of Medicine,* 1986, 60:194–208; S. Rothman, *Woman's Proper Place: A History of Changing Practices, 1870 to the Present* (New York: Basic Books, 1978); W. L. O'Neill, *Everyone Was Brave: A History of Feminism in America* (New York: Quadrangle, New York Times Books, 1974); K. J. Blair, *The Clubwoman as Feminist: True Womanhood Redefined, 1868–1914* (New York: Holmes and Meier Publishers, 1980).

6. J. W. Ballantyne, "The Nature of Pregnancy and Its Practical Bearings," *British Medical Journal,* February 1914, 14:349–355; L. G. Miller, "Pain, Parturition, and the Profession: Twilight Sleep in America," in *Health Care in America: Essays in Social His-*

tory, edited by S. Reverby and D. Rosner (Philadelphia: Temple University Press, 1979), pp. 19-44.

7. Tracy and Leupp.

8. R. K. Carter, *The Sleeping Car "Twilight," or Motherhood Without Pain* (Boston: Chapple Publishing, 1915), p. 176.

9. Here are the years of the founding of several American women's colleges: Mount Holyoke, 1837; Columbia (S.C.), 1854; Queens, 1857; Vassar, 1861; Smith, 1875; Bryn Mawr, 1880; Converse, 1889; Salem, 1889; Meredith, 1891; Randolph Macon, 1891; Sweet Briar, 1901.

10. W. H. W. Knipe, "The Freiburg Method of Dämmerschlaf or Twilight Sleep," *American Journal of Obstetrics and Gynecology,* 1914, 70:884-909.

11. M. Tracy and M. Boyd, *Painless Childbirth* (New York: Frederick A. Stokes, 1915), pp. xxx-xxxiii; H. Rion, *The Truth About Twilight Sleep* (New York: McBride, Nast, 1915); G. H. Davis, *Painless Childbirth: Eutocia and Nitrous Oxide-Oxygen Analgesia* (Chicago: Forbes, 1916); M. C. Stopes, *Radiant Motherhood: A Book for Those Who Are Creating the Future* (London: G. P. Putnam's Sons, 1925); B. Van Hoosen, *Scopolamine-Morphine Anaesthesia* (Chicago: House of Manz, 1915); A. M. Hellman, *Amnesia and Analgesia in Parturition (Twilight Sleep)* (New York: Paul B. Hoeber, 1915).

12. Miller; M. Sandelowski, *Pain, Pleasure, and American Childbirth: From the Twilight Sleep to the Read Method, 1914-1960* (Westport, Conn.: Greenwood Press, 1984); "Authority Spoke Too Soon!" *New York Times,* August 24, 1914; "Accusing the Medical Profession," *New York Times,* September 17, 1914; "An Answer Hardly Adequate," *New York Times,* September 22, 1914; "Twilight Sleep Vindicated," *New York Times,* October 20, 1914; "Twilight Sleep Once More," *New York Times,* November 7, 1914; "They Do So Hate Coercion!" *New York Times,* November 30, 1914; "A Story of Ethics Violated," *New York Times,* February 5, 1915; "Spoiling a Frank Admission," *New York Times,* April 5, 1915.

13. Tracy and Boyd, pp. xxx-xxxiii; Davis; C. Leupp and B. Hendricks, "Twilight Sleep," *McClure's Magazine,* April 1915, pp. 25-37.

14. B. Krönig, "The Difference Between the Older and the

Newer Treatments of X-Ray and Radium in Gynecological Diseases,"
Surgery, Gynecology, and Obstetrics, 1914, 18:529–532.

15. "Twilight Sleep Is Successful in 120 Cases Here," *New York
Times,* August 30, 1914; G. Ginsberg, "Twilight Sleep: Physician Who
Observed It Closely Condemns the Treatment," *New York Times,*
September 20, 1914; C. J. Gauss, "Anwendung des Skopolamin-
Morphium Dämmerschlafes in der Geburtshilfe," *Medizinische
Klinik,* 1906, 2:136–138.

16. J. W. Williams, *Obstetrics,* 2d ed. (New York: Appleton,
1908), p. 324; J. DeLee, *The Principles and Practice of Obstetrics*
(Philadelphia: W. B. Saunders, 1918), pp. 303–307; "A Special Discussion with Reference to 'Twilight Sleep' by the Request of the
Committee on Public Health, Hospitals and Budget of the Academy
for a Formal Expression on This Subject," *American Journal of
Obstetrics,* 1915, 71:332–344.

17. D. Caton, "In the Present State of Our Knowledge: Early
Use of Opioids in Obstetrics," *Anesthesiology,* 1985, 82:779–784;
J. Pereira, *The Elements of Materia Medica and Therapeutics*
(London: Longman, Brown, Green and Longmans, 1842), pp.
1755–1758; S. Crumpe, *An Inquiry into the Nature and Prop-
erties of Opium* (London: G. G. and J. Robinson, 1793), pp.
23–97; R. Dunglison, *General Therapeutics and Materia Medica*
(Philadelphia: Lea and Blanchard, 1843), pp. 318-340; C. Binz,
Lectures on Pharmacology, translated by A. C. Latham (London:
New Sydenham Society, 1895), 1:47–67; T. L. Brunton, *A Text
Book of Pharmacology, Therapeutics and Materia Medica,* 3d ed.
(London: Macmillan, 1887), p. 854.

18. Today, uterine rupture is an indication for immediate surgery. Before anesthesia, however, this was not an option. The only
way physicians could give the uterus time to heal was to allow it to
"rest," that is, be free of contractions for a period of time. To stop
contractions they gave morphine (Pereira).

19. C. Sherrington, *The Integrative Action of the Nervous
System* (New Haven: Yale University Press, 1961).

20. J. W. Comfort, *Thompsonian Practice of Midwifery and
Treatment of Complaints Peculiar to Women and Children* (Philadelphia: A. Comfort, 1845); W. H. Howell, *A Text Book of Physiology,* 7th ed. (Philadelphia: W. B. Saunders, 1919), p. 998; M. Fos-

ter, *Physiology* (London: Macmillan, 1879), pp. 621–630; Williams, p. 324.

21. J. W. Williams, *Obstetrics* (New York: D. Appleton, 1903), pp. 291–294; Williams, *Obstetrics* (1908); Pereira; Crumpe; Dunglison; Binz; Brunton; Sherrington; Howell, *A Text Book of Physiology*, 7th ed. (Philadelphia: W. B. Saunders, 1919), p. 998; Foster; Williams, *Obstetrics* (1903); W. Tyler-Smith, *Parturition and the Principles and Practice of Obstetrics* (London: John Churchill, 1849), pp. 213–226.

22. A. Routh, "Parturition During Paraplegia, with Cases," *Transactions of the Obstetrical Society of London*, 1897, 39:191–229; N. M. Gertsman, "Über Uterusinnervation an Hand des Falles einer Geburt bei Querschnittslähmung," *Monatsschrift Geburtshilfe Gynäkologie*, 1926, 73:73, 253–257; O. Kreis, "Über Medullarnarkose bei Gebärenden," *Centralblatt Gynäkologie*, 1900, 28: 724–727; D. I. Macht, "History of Opium and Some of the Preparations and Alkaloids," *Journal of the American Medical Association*, 1915, 64:477–481.

23. Williams, *Obstetrics* (1903).

24. P. C. Barker, "Concerning the Action of Opium upon the Uterus and Particularly as a Parturient Agent," *New York Medical Journal*, 1869, 9:261–268; H. Hensen, "Über den Einfluss des Morphiums und des Aethers auf die Wehenthätigkeit des Uterus," *Archiv für Gynäkologie*, 1898, 55:129–177.

25. Tyler-Smith, pp. 213–226.

26. Pereira.

27. W. T. Lusk, "Morphia in Childbirth," *American Journal of Obstetrical Disease of Women and Children*, 1877, 10:612–623; W. Hale-White, *Textbook of Pharmacology and Therapeutics* (Edinburgh: Adam and Charles Black, 1901), p. 240; B. Cook-Hirst, *A Textbook of Obstetrics* (Philadelphia: W. B. Saunders, 1913), pp. 187–189, 303–304.

28. "Doctors Disagree on Twilight Sleep," *New York Times*, August 24, 1915; "Mrs. Francis X. Carmody Buried," *New York Times*, August 25, 1915.

29. "Proclaiming a Poor Triumph," *New York Times*, August 25, 1915; "To Fight Twilight Sleep," *New York Times*, August 31, 1915.

30. W. Aranow, "A Post Mortem on Twilight Sleep," *New York*

Medical Journal, 1918, 108:64–66; C. J. Gauss, "Twenty-Five Years of Obstetrical Analgesia," *British Journal of Anaesthesia,* 1929, 6: 139–148.

Chapter Nine
The National Birthday Trust Fund Campaign in Great Britain

1. Pamphlet, May 4, 1948 (National Birthday Trust Fund 51/G4/3/1); pamphlet, "A Brief Account of the Fund's Activities, November 12, 1953" (National Birthday Trust Fund 51/G5/5). The numbers in these and subsequent references in this chapter refer to the locations of documents in the Archives of the National Birthday Trust Fund (hereafter NBTF), now in the library of the Wellcome Institute for the History of Medicine, London. Material from the NBTF Archives is reproduced by permission of Wellbeing and the Wellcome Institute.

2. "Relief of Pain in Childbirth, 1948" (NBTF 51/G4/3/1).

3. J. S. Mill, "The Subjection of Women," in *On Liberty, with the Subjection of Women and Chapters on Socialism,* edited by S. Collini (Cambridge: Cambridge University Press, 1989), pp. 119–217.

4. V. Brittain, *Testament of Experience* ([New York]: Wideview Books, 1970), pp. 51–52.

5. Joint Committee of the Royal College of Obstetricians and Gynaecologists and the Population Investigation Committee, *Maternity in Great Britain* (London: Oxford University Press, 1948), pp. 28–77, 81, 80, 83, 611; J. W. Leavitt, "Joseph B. DeLee and the Practice of Preventive Obstetrics," *American Journal of Public Health,* 1988, 78:1353–1359.

6. J. B. DeLee, "The Prophylactic Forceps Operation," *American Journal of Obstetric Gynecology,* 1920, 1:34–44.

7. A. Flint, "Responsibility of the Medical Profession in Further Reducing Maternal Mortality," *American Journal of Obstetric Gynecology,* 1925, 19:864–866; G. J. Engelmann, "Birth and Death Rate as Influenced by Obstetric and Gynecic Progress," *Boston Medicine and Surgery Journal,* 1902, 146:505–508, 541–544; W. E. Studiford, "The Relation of Obstetrics to Preventive Medicine," *Boston Medicine and Surgery Journal,* 1924, 191:617–630.

8. C. H. Davis, "Discussion on Anesthesia," *Journal of the American Medical Association,* 1923, 81:1095-1096; C. M. Steer, "Obstetrics at Sloane—Then and Now," *Obstetric and Gynecology Survey,* 1954, 9:631-644; I. Loudon, *Death in Childbirth: An International Study of Maternal Care and Maternal Mortality, 1800-1950* (Oxford: Clarendon Press, 1992), pp. 187, 220-223, 172-233, 216-232; A. M. Claye, "Anaesthesia and Analgesia in Normal Labour Cases: One Year's Experience at a Maternity Hospital," *Lancet,* 1932, 223:180-182.

9. Brittain; V. Woolf, *Three Guineas* (London: Hogarth Press, 1943), p. 124; J. Lewis, "Mothers and Maternal Policies in the Twentieth Century," in *The Politics of Maternity Care: Services for Childbearing Women in Twentieth-Century Britain,* edited by J. Garcia, R. Kilpatrick, and M. Richards (Oxford: Clarendon Paperbacks, 1990), pp. 15-29.

10. Public Health Department, *Report of London County Council, 1932, by Letitia Fairfield, CBE, MD, Chb, DPH, Senior Medical Officer* (NBTF 42/F7/4).

11. *The National Birthday Trust Fund History, 1955* (NBTF 51/G5/5); S. K. Kent, *Sex and Suffrage in Britain, 1860-1914* (Princeton: Princeton University Press, 1987), pp. 157-183.

12. A. Edwards, "Mothers Should Make a Fuss," *Daily Express,* February 12, 1946; "We've Changed Our Minds About Having Babies," *Daily Mirror* (London), May 17, 1945, p. 7.

13. "Mothers Want the Princess' Drugs," *Evening Standard* (London), November 15, 1948; Woolf, *Three Guineas,* p. 293.

14. *Wife and Citizen: A Journal Advocating the Economic and Social Emancipation of All Women,* November 1945, 6(11); Edwards.

15. *A Brief Account of the Trust's Activities, November 12, 1953* (NBTF 51/G4/4).

16. D. Baird, "The Evolution of Modern Obstetrics," *Lancet,* 1960, 2:557-564, 609-614; Loudon.

17. "Recent Advances in Obstetrics," *Lancet,* 1926, 210:241; H. Jellett, "The Future of Obstetrical Practice," *Lancet,* 1929, 217:859-964; "The Teaching of Obstetrics," *Lancet,* 1932, 222:1201-1202.

18. Loudon.

19. "Chloroform Capsules," *Lancet*, 1932, 223:1015; J. Cahn, "Chloroform Capsules in Childbirth," letter to the editor, *Lancet*, 1932, 223:1024.

20. G. F. Marx and T. Katsnelson, "The Introduction of Nitrous Oxide Analgesia into Obstetrics," *Obstetric Gynecology*, 1992, 80: 715-718; W. D. A. Smith, *Under the Influence: A History of Nitrous Oxide and Oxygen Anaesthesia* (Park Ridge, Ill.: Wood Library-Museum of Anesthesiology, 1982).

21. R. J. Minnitt, "Self-Administered Analgesia for the Midwifery of General Practice," *Proceedings of the Royal Society of Medicine*, 1934, 27:1313-1318; R. J. Minnitt, "A New Technique for the Self-Administration of Gas-Air Analgesia in Labour," *Lancet*, 1934, 226:1278-1279; J. Elam, "Gas-and-Air Apparatus for Midwives," *Lancet*, 1935, 30:1253-1254; J. Elam, "Analgesia in Domiciliary Midwifery," *Journal of Obstetric Gynecology of the British Empire*, 46(1):61-70.

22. H. Roberts and others, "Effects of Some Analgesic Drugs Used in Childbirth," *Lancet*, 1957, 19:128-132; *A Brief Account of the Fund's Activities, November 12, 1953* (NBTF 51/G5/5).

23. "Midwives and the Use of Drugs," *Lancet*, 1932, 223:191-192; *Report on the Work of the Central Midwives Board for the Years 1955 and 1961* (NBTF 51/G4/3/1); K. Kane, "Analgesia During Labour," *Midwives Chronicle and Nursing Notes*, February 1951, pp. 42-46.

24. Minnitt's opinion of hypoxia was different from that of present-day obstetricians. He wrote, "Cyanosis of the mother was rather encouraged, and indeed, in one case actually produced, in order that the delivery could be accomplished by forceps" (Minnitt, "Self-Administered Analgesia").

25. *Resolution of the Maternity and Child Welfare Committee of the Hertfordshire County Council, Relief of Sufferings in Childbirth, October 4, 1934* (NBTF 44/F10/1/1).

26. "We've Changed Our Minds About Having Babies."

27. Joint Committee; K. K. Conrad, "Pain in Childbirth: Report of the Subcommittee of the Medical Women's Federation," *British Medical Journal*, February 1949, 1:333-337; "The Pain of Labour," *Lancet*, 1939, 236:888-891.

28. W. C. Danforth and C. H. Davis, "Obstetric Analgesia and

Anesthesia: A Consideration of Nitrous Oxide-Oxygen and Various Combined Methods," *Journal of the American Medical Association*, 1923, 81:1090-1096.

29. "Midwives and the Use of Drugs," *Lancet*, 1932, 223: 191-192.

30. F. Roques, "Anaesthesia for Eutocia," *Lancet*, 1933, 224: 177-182; M. P. Rucker, "The Use of Novocaine in Obstetrics," *American Journal of Obstetrics and Gynecology*, 1925, 35:35-47; H. Schlimpert, "Concerning Sacral Anaesthesia," *Surgery, Gynecology, and Obstetrics*, 1913, 16:488-493; S. P. Oldham, "Sacral Anesthesia in Obstetrics," *American Journal of Surgery*, 1925, 39: 42-45; R. A. Hingson and W. B. Edwards, "Continuous Caudal Analgesia: An Analysis of the First Ten Thousand Confinements Thus Managed with the Report of the Authors' First Thousand Cases," *Journal of the American Medical Association*, 1942, 123:538-546; R. Goltz, "Über den Einfluss des Nervensystems auf die Vorgänge während der Schwangerschaft und des Gebäraks," *Archiv für des Gestational Physiologie*, 1874, 9:552-565; J. N. Langley and H. K. Anderson, "The Innervation of the Pelvic and Adjoining Viscera," *Journal of Physiology*, 1895-1896, 19:71-139; R. J. Behan, *Pain: Its Origin, Conduction, Perception and Diagnostic Significance* (New York: D. Appleton, 1917), pp. 705-740.

31. H. Schwarz, "Painless Childbirth and the Safe Conduct of Labor," *American Journal of Obstetrics and Gynecology*, 1919, 79: 46-62.

32. J. W. Williams, "The Prophylactic Forceps Operation," *American Journal of Obstetrics and Gynecology*, 1920, 15:77-84; R. W. Holmes, "The Fad and Fancies of Obstetrics: A Comment on the Pseudoscientific Trend of Modern Obstetrics," *American Journal of Obstetrics and Gynecology*, 1921, 16:225-237; J. Young, "Maternal Mortality and Maternal Mortality Rates," *American Journal of Obstetrics and Gynecology*, 1936, 31:198-212.

33. Joint Committee.

Chapter Ten
Grantly Dick Read and the Natural Childbirth Movement

1. G. D. Read, *Childbirth Without Fear* (London: Heinemann, 1954).

2. G. D. Read, *Unpublished Autobiography* (Installment 5, p. 16, Grantly Dick Read 9 A/92); G. D. Read, *Natural Childbirth* (London: Heinemann, 1933), pp. 86, 37-38, 42-45, vii; G. D. Read, *Account of Visit to USA, 1958* (pp. 42-45, Grantly Dick Read 10 F/107). The numbers in these and other references in this chapter describe the locations of documents in the Grantly Dick Read archives, hereafter GDR, in the library of the Wellcome Institute for the History of Medicine, London. Material from the GDR archives is reproduced by permission of Laurence Pollinger Limited and the Estate of Dr. Grantly Dick Read.

3. G. D. Read, *Revelation of Childbirth* (London: Heinemann, 1943), pp. 41-52, 105; Read, *Natural Childbirth;* Read, *Account of Visit to USA.*

4. Read, *Natural Childbirth.*

5. Read, *Revelation of Childbirth;* G. D. Read, *Childbirth Without Fear* (New York: Harper and Row, 1959), pp. 63, 64-65, 143, 105, 197-202: G. D. Read, *Lecture Notes: London Hospital Medical Society, October 5, 1954* (GDR 23 C/42); V. Brittain, *Honourable Estate* (New York: Macmillan, 1936).

6. Read, *Natural Childbirth;* Read, *Revelation of Childbirth.*

7. J. Read, *Lecture Notes, First International Congress for the Release of Tensions and Re-Education of Functional Movement, Copenhagen, Denmark, July 30, 1959* (GDR 9 A/89).

8. G. D. Read, *Letter to His Mother, June 16, 1938* (GDR 10 A/95); Read, *Childbirth Without Fear.*

9. G. D. Read, *Unpublished Autobiography* (Installment 2, p. 24, GDR 9 A/92).

10. *News Chronicle, January 20, 1956* (GDR 22 C/33); Read, *Natural Childbirth.*

11. G. D. Read, *Typewritten Notes, 1944-45* (GDR 14 B/13); G. D. Read, *Lecture Notes, University of Witwatersrand, October 11, 1949* (GDR 27 C/76).

12. Read, *Account of Visit to USA*, pp. 40–42; Read, *Childbirth Without Fear.*

13. T. Denman, *An Introduction to the Practice of Midwifery* (London: E. Cox, 1832), p. 235; S. Bard, *A Compendium on the Theory and Practice of Midwifery Containing Practical Instructions for the Management of Women During Pregnancy, in Labor and in Child-Bed* (New York: Collins, 1812), p. 122.

14. D. Caton, "Obstetric Anesthesia: The First Ten Years," *Anesthesiology,* 1970, 33:102–109; R. W. Holmes, "The Fads and Fancies of Obstetrics: A Comment on the Pseudoscientific Trend of Modern Obstetrics," *American Journal of Obstetrics and Gynecology,* 1921, 2:224–237; J. B. DeLee, "The Prophylactic Forceps Operation," *American Journal of Obstetrics and Gynecology,* 1920, 1:34–44, 77–84.

15. Obituary of G. D. Read, *British Medical Journal,* 1959; L. J. Clewin, *London Medical Gazette* (London), September 1957.

16. G. D. Read, *Letter to B. W. Williams, February 8, 1949* (GDR 53 L/190).

17. Read, *Account of Visit to USA;* Read, *Revelation of Childbirth;* G. D. Read, *Lecture: The Divine Healing Principle in Childbirth, November 1955* (GDR 22 C/33); G. D. Read, *Lecture Notes, Middlesex Hospital Medical Society, March 10, 1947* (GDR 25 C/72).

18. Read, *Revelation of Childbirth;* G. D. Read, "Correlation of Physical and Emotional Phenomena of Natural Labor," *Journal of Obstetrical Gynaecology, British Empire,* 1946, 53:55–61; Read, *Childbirth Without Fear.*

19. G. D. Read, "Article," in *The People* (Petersfield), February 13, 1956.

20. G. D. Read, *Motherhood in the Post War World* (London: Heinemann, 1944), pp. 15–16.

21. N. Eastman, *Letter to GDR, June 9, 1943* (GDR 53 L/195); N. Eastman, "Editorial Comments," *Obstetric Gynecology Survey,* 1946, 1:459; H. Thoms and R. H. Wyatt, "A Natural Childbirth Program," *American Journal of Public Health,* 1950, 40:787–791.

22. T. Deighton, *Letter to Miss Riddick, May 9, 1957* (National Birthday Trust Fund 44 F/10/6); C. L. Beynon, "Whither Natural Childbirth?" *British Medical Journal,* 1955, p. 475; "A Harley Street

Gynecologist," letter to the editor, *The People,* January 15, 1956; H. Roberts, letter to the editor, *Briefs of the Maternity Center Association of NY,* November 17, 1953.

23. D. Reid and M. E. Cohen, "Trends in Obstetrics," *Journal of the American Medical Association,* 1950, 142:615–623; N. Eastman, "Editorial," *Obstetric Gynecology Survey,* 1951, 6:163–167.

24. Read, *Childbirth Without Fear;* G. D. Read, Letter, January 8, 1949 (GDR d.150).

25. A. Flint, "Responsibility of the Medical Profession in Further Reducing Maternal Mortality," *American Journal of Obstetric Gynecology,* 1925, 9:864–866; *Wife and Citizen: A Journal Advocating the Economic and Social Emancipation of All Women,* November 1945, 6(11) (GDR 58 D/272).

26. P. Buck, *The Good Earth* (New York: John Day, 1931), pp. 35–48; D. Lessing, *Children of Violence: A Proper Marriage* (New York: Simon and Schuster, 1970), pp. 137–147; M. McCarthy, *The Group* (London: Harcourt Brace, 1963); S. Plath, *The Bell Jar* (New York: Harper and Row, 1975), pp. 52–55.

27. G. D. Read, *Personal Notes, October 10, 1958* (GDR 22 C/33).

28. F. Lamaze, *Painless Childbirth: Psychoprophylactic Method,* translated by L. R. Celestin (London: Burke, 1956); P. Vellay, *Childbirth Without Pain,* translated by D. Lloyd (London: Hutchinson, 1959); M. Karmel, *Thank You Dr. Lamaze: A Mother's Experiences in Painless Childbirth* (Philadelphia: J. B. Lippincott, 1959).

29. G. D. Read, *Unpublished Notes* (GDR 22 C/33); Read, "Article" (1956).

30. *New York Times,* January 9, 1956.

31. *Irish News* (Belfast), January 9, 1956; *Washington Post* (Washington, D.C.), January 9, 1956; *News Chronicle* (London), January 9, 1956; *News Chronicle* (London), January 10, 1956.

32. *New York Times,* January 9, 1956.

33. A. N. Thomas, *Doctor Courageous: The Story of Grantly Dick Read* (London: Heinemann, 1957), p. 76.

34. J. Duns, *Memoir of Sir James Y. Simpson, Bart.* (Edinburgh: Edmonston and Douglas, 1873), p. 106.

35. R. P. Lederman and others, "The Relationship of Maternal Anxiety, Plasma Catecholamines and Plasma Cortisol to Progress

in Labor," *American Journal of Obstetric Gynecology*, 1978, 132: 495–500; F. P. Zuspan, L. A. Cibils, and S. V. Pose, "Myometrial and Cardiovascular Responses to Alterations in Plasma Epinephrine and Norepinephrine," *American Journal of Obstetrics and Gynecology*, 1962, 84:841–851; J. Kennell and others, "Continuous Emotional Support During Labor in a U.S. Hospital: A Randomized Controlled Trial," *Journal of the American Medical Association*, 1991, 265: 2197–2201; J. R. Scott and N. B. Rose, "Effect of Psychoprophylaxis (Lamaze Preparation) on Labor and Delivery in Primiparas," *New England Journal of Medicine*, 1976, 294:1205–1207; W. L. Wolman and others, "Postpartum Depression and Companionship in the Clinical Birth Environment: A Randomized Controlled Study," *American Journal of Obstetric Gynecology*, 1993, 168:1388–1399.

36. F. Slaughter, "To Ease the Pangs," *New York Times*, October 6, 1957.

Chapter Eleven
The Danger of Drugs and the Social Value of Pain

1. J. T. Gwathmey and others, "Painless Childbirth by Synergistic Methods," *American Journal of Obstetric Gynecology*, 1923, 6:456.

2. J. Snow, "On the Administration of Chloroform During Parturition," *London Association Medical Journal*, 1853, p. 500; J. Snow, "On Asphyxia and on the Resuscitation of Stillborn Children'" *London Medical Gazette*, 1841–1842, pp. 222–227; E. Döbeli, "Über die Empfindlichkeit verschieden alter Tiere gegen die Opiumalkaloide," *Monatsschrift für Kinderheilkunde*, 1911, 9: 397–420; N. B. Eddy, "The Variation with Age in the Toxic Effects of Morphine, Codeine, and Some of Their Derivatives," *Journal of Pharmacology*, 1930, 66:182–201; H. A. Schlossmann, "The Relationship Between Age and the Action of Atropine and Morphine," *Journal of Pharmacology*, 1937, 60:14–31.

3. S. H. Calmes, "Virginia Apgar: A Woman Physician's Career in a Developing Specialty," *Journal of the American Medical Woman's Association*, 1984, 39:184–188; S. H. Calmes, "Development of the Apgar Score," in *Proceedings of the First International Symposium on Anesthesia*, edited by J. Ruprecht, M. J. Lieburg, and J. A. Lee

(Berlin: Springer-Verlag, 1985), pp. 45-48; V. Apgar, "Proposal for a New Method of Evaluation of Newborn Infants," *Anesthesia and Analgesia,* 1953, 32:260-267; V. Apgar and others, "Comparison of Regional and General Anesthesia in Obstetrics with Special Reference to Transmission of Cyclopropane Across the Placenta," *Journal of the American Medical Association,* 1957, 165:2155-2161.

4. L. S. James and others, "Acid-Base Status of Human Infants in Relation to Birth Asphyxia and Onset of Respiration," *Journal of Pediatrics,* 1958, 52:379-394; B. Pasamanick and A. M. Lilienfeld, "Association of Maternal and Fetal Factors with Development of Mental Deficiency," *Journal of the American Medical Association,* 1955, 159:155-160; F. Schreiber, "Apnea of the Newborn and Associated Cerebral Injury," *Journal of the American Medical Association,* 1938, 111:1263-1268.

5. J. Mayow, quoted in J. Needham, *Chemical Embryology* (New York: Hafner Publishing, 1963), p. 173; D. H. Barron, "A History of Fetal Respiration: From Harvey's Question (1651) to Zweifel's Answer (1876)," in *Fetal and Newborn Cardiovascular Physiology,* vol. 1: *Developmental Aspects,* edited by L. D. Longo and D. D. Reneau (New York: Garland STPM Press, 1978), pp. 1-32.

6. K. J. Anselmino and F. Hoffman, "Die Ursachen des Icterus Neonatorum," *Archiv für Gynaekologie,* 1930, 143:477-499; J. Barcroft, "The Conditions of Fetal Respiration," *Lancet,* 1933, 225: 1021-1024; N. J. Eastman, "Foetal Blood Studies, I. The Oxygen Relationships of Umbilical Cord Blood at Birth," *Bulletin of Johns Hopkins Hospital,* 1930, 47:221-230; J. Barcroft, *Researches on Pre-Natal Life* (Oxford: Basil Blackwell, 1946); E. S. Taylor, G. D. Govan, and W. C. Scott, "Oxygen Saturation of the Blood of the Newborn, as Affected by Maternal Anesthetic Agents," *American Journal of Obstetric Gynecology,* 1951, 61:840-854; H. Henderson, R. Mosher, and N. M. Bittrich, "Oxygen Studies of the Cord Blood of Caesarean-Born Infants," *American Journal of Obstetric Gynecology,* 1957, 74:654-676; C. A. Smith, "Effect of Obstetrical Anesthesia upon Oxygenation of Maternal and Fetal Blood with Particular Reference to Cyclopropane," *Surgery, Gynecology, and Obstetrics,* 1939, 69:584-593; P. Lund, "Influence of Anesthesia on Infant Mortality Rate in Caesarean Section," *Journal of the American Medical Association,* 1955, 159:1586-1591.

7. I. Loudon, *Death in Childbirth: An International Study of Maternal Care and Maternal Mortality, 1800-1950* (New York: Oxford University Press, 1992), pp. 542-582.

8. D. H. Barron and others, "Adaptions of Pregnant Ewes and Their Fetuses to High Altitude," in *Symposium on the Physiological Effects of High Altitude* (Oxford: Pergamon Press, 1963), pp. 115-129.

9. Eddy.

10. T. B. Brazelton, "Effect of Prenatal Drugs on the Behavior of the Neonate," *American Journal of Psychiatry*, 1970, 126: 1261-1266; D. B. Rosenblatt and others, "The Influence of Maternal Analgesia on Neonatal Behaviour, II. Epidural Bupivacaine," *British Journal of Obstetrics and Gynaecology*, 1981, 88:407; J. W. Scanlon, W. U. Brown, and J. B. Weiss, "Neurobehavioral Responses of Newborn Infants After Maternal Epidural Anesthesia," *Anesthesiology*, 1974, 40:121-128.

11. Rosenblatt and others.

12. R. Nisbet, *History of the Idea of Progress* (New York: Basic Books, 1980), pp. 317-350.

13. G. D. Read, *Motherhood in the Post War World* (London: Heinemann, 1944), pp. 15-16.

14. B. Spock, *The Common Sense Book of Baby and Child Care* (New York: Duel, Sloan and Pearce, 1945), p. 3; Scanlon, Brown, and Weiss.

15. A. E. Bernstein, *The Formation of Hell: Death and Retribution in the Ancient and Early Christian Worlds* (Ithaca: Cornell University Press, 1993); Homer, *The Iliad*, translated by R. Fagles (New York: Viking, 1990), book I, ll. 10-120; book II, ll. 313-318; J. H. Langbein, *Torture and the Law of Proof: Europe and England in the Ancient Régime* (Chicago: University of Chicago Press, 1977); P. Spierenburg, *The Spectacle of Suffering: Executions and the Evolution of Repression: From a Preindustrial Metropolis to the European Experience* (New York: Cambridge University Press, 1984); E. Scarry, *The Body in Pain: The Making and Unmaking of the World* (New York: Oxford University Press, 1985); R. MacMullen, *Christianizing the Roman Empire (A.D. 100-400)* (New Haven: Yale University Press, 1984); W. A. Meeks, *The First Urban

Christians: The Social World of the Apostle Paul (New Haven: Yale University Press, 1983); Aeschylus, *Oresteia,* translated by R. Fitzgerald (New York: Doubleday, 1962), p. 2; N. Malebranche, *The Search After Truth (and) Elucidations of the Search After Truth,* translated by T. M. Lennon and P. J. Olscamp (Columbus: Ohio State University Press, 1980), p. 129; J. Locke, *An Essay Concerning Human Understanding* (Great Britain: J. M. Dent and Sons, 1947), p. 41; J. Bentham, *An Introduction to the Principles of Morals and Legislation,* edited by J. H. Burns, J. H. Hart, and H. L. A. Hart (New York: Methuen, 1982).

16. M. Cohen, *The Philosophy of John Stuart Mill: Ethical, Political and Religious* (New York: Random House, 1961); D. Caton, "The Poem in the Pain: The Social Significance of Pain in Western Civilization," *Anesthesiology,* 1994, 81:1044–1052; G. Himmerfarb, *Poverty and Compassion: The Moral Imagination of the Late Victorians* (New York: Knopf, 1984); M. Ignatieff, *A Just Measure of Pain: The Penitentiary in the Industrial Revolution, 1750–1850* (New York: Pantheon Books, 1978); N. Frye, *Anatomy of Criticism* (Princeton: Princeton University Press, 1973), p. 207.

17. E. Hemingway, "The Snows of Kilimanjaro," in *The Complete Short Stories of Ernest Hemingway,* edited by F. Vagia (New York: Schreibner Press, 1987), p. 3; C. Baker, *Ernest Hemingway: Selected Letters, 1917–1961* (New York: Schreibner Press, 1981), p. 408; R. Wright, *Black Boy* (New York: Harper and Row, 1989), p. 112; W. Percy, *Love in the Ruins: The Adventures of a Bad Catholic at a Time near the End of the World* (New York: Dell, 1972), p. 188; W. Percy, *The Moviegoer* (New York: Avon Books, 1982); W. Stegner, *All the Little Live Things* (New York: Penguin Books, 1967), pp. 297–298.

18. G. Greene, *The Power and the Glory* (New York: Bantam Books, 1968), pp. 64, 184.

19. Stegner.

20. C. E. Rosenberg, *The Care of Strangers: The Rise of America's Hospital System* (New York: Basic Books, 1987), pp. 206–236.

21. Joint Committee of the Royal College of Obstetricians and Gynaecologists and the Population Investigation Committee, *Ma-*

ternity in Great Britain (London: Oxford University Press, 1948), p. 61; D. Lessing, *A Proper Marriage* (New York: Plume, 1952), pp. 140-154.

22. L. T. Ulrich, *A Midwife's Tale: The Life of Martha Ballard Based on Her Diary, 1785-1812* (New York: Knopf), p. 183.

23. J. S. Lewis, *In the Family Way: Childbearing in the British Aristocracy, 1760-1860* (New Brunswick, N.J.: Rutgers University Press, 1986).

24. Euripides, *Medea*, in *Euripides' Ten Plays*, edited by M. Hadas and J. McLean (New York: Dial Press, 1979), p. 38; Homer, *Iliad*, book II, pp. 313-318; H. King, "The Early Anodynes: Pain in the Ancient World," in *The History of the Management of Pain: From Early Principles to Present Practice*, edited by R. D. Mann (Camforth: Parthenon Publishing Group, 1988), pp. 51-62.

25. R. P. Lederman and others, "The Relationship of Maternal Anxiety, Plasma Catecholamines, and Plasma Cortisol to Progress in Labor," *American Journal of Obstetric Gynecology*, 1978, 132: 495-500; F. P. Zuspan, L. A. Cibils and S. V. Pose, "Myometrial and Cardiovascular Responses to Alterations in Plasma Epinephrine and Norepinephrine," *American Journal of Obstetrics and Gynecology*, 1962, 84:841-851; J. Kennell and others, "Continuous Emotional Support During Labor in a U.S. Hospital: A Randomized Controlled Trial," *Journal of the American Medical Association*, 1919, 265: 2197-2201; J. R. Scott and N. N. Rose, "Effect of Psychoprophylaxis (Lamaze Preparation) on Labor and Delivery in Primiparas," *New England Journal of Medicine*, 1976, 294:1205-1207; G. D. Read, "Correlation of Physical and Emotional Phenomena of Natural Labour," *Journal of Obstetrics and Gynaecology, British Empire*, 1946, 53:55-61; W. L. Wolman and others, "Postpartum Depression and Companionship in the Clinical Birth Environment: A Randomized, Controlled Study," *American Journal of Obstetric Gynecology*, 1993, 168:1388-1393.

26. P. Simkin, *The Birth Partner* (Boston: Harvard Common Press, 1989); P. Perez and C. Snedeker, *Special Women: The Role of the Professional Labor Assistant* (Seattle: Penny Press, 1990); M. H. Klaus, J. H. Kennell, and P. H. Klaus, *Mothering the Mother* (Reading, Penn.: Addison-Wesley, 1993), p. 3.

Chapter Twelve
Current Controversy

1. S. K. Kent, *Sex and Suffrage in Britain, 1860-1914* (Princeton: Princeton University Press, 1987), pp. 119-139; W. W. Wertz and D. C. Wertz, *Lying-In: A History of Childbirth in America* (New York: Schocken Books, 1979), pp. 109-119, 143, 145; P. S. Eakins, *The American Way of Birth* (Philadelphia: Temple University Press, 1986); J. W. Leavitt, *Brought to Bed: Childbearing in America, 1750-1950* (Oxford: Oxford University Press, 1986), pp. 134-141, 170-212; A. Oakley, *The Captured Womb: A History of the Medical Care of Pregnant Women* (Oxford: Basil Blackwell, 1984); M. Sandelowski, *Pain, Pleasure and American Childbirth: From the Twilight Sleep to the Read Method, 1914-1960* (London: Greenwood Press, 1984), pp. 60-71; S. Arms, *Immaculate Deception: A New Look at Women and Childbirth in America* (Boston: Houghton Mifflin, 1975).

2. Wertz and Wertz; W. R. Arney, *Power and the Profession of Obstetrics* (Chicago: University of Chicago Press, 1983), pp. 20-50; B. K. Rothman, "The Social Construction of Birth," in *The American Way of Birth*, edited by P. S. Eakins (Philadelphia: Temple University Press, 1986), p. 104; E. W. Schuarz, "The Engineering of Childbirth: A New Obstetric Programme as Reflected in British Obstetric Textbooks, 1960-1980," in *The Politics of Maternity Care*, edited by J. Garcia, R. Kilpatrick, and M. Richards (Oxford: Clarendon Press, 1990), p. 57: Leavitt.

3. C. E. Rosenberg, *The Care of Strangers: The Rise of America's Hospital System* (New York: Basic Books, 1987).

4. K. K. Conrad, "Pain in Childbirth: Report of the Subcommittee of the Medical Women's Federation," *British Medical Journal*, February 26, 1949, pp. 333-337; Joint Committee of the Royal College of Obstetricians and Gynaecologists and the Population Investigation Committee, *Maternity in Great Britain.* (London: Oxford University Press, 1948), pp. 55-66.

5. R. J. Behan, *Pain* (New York: Century Appleton, 1915), p. 18; C. Sherrington, *The Integrative Action of the Nervous System* (New Haven: Yale University Press, 1961), p. 229.

6. M. Kaufman, *American Medical Education: The Formative Years, 1765-1910* (Westport, Conn.: Greenwood Press, 1976).

7. E. Dickinson, *The Complete Poems of Emily Dickinson,* edited by T. H. Johnson (Boston: Little, Brown, 1960), pp. 162, 323; V. S. Naipaul, *A Bend in the River* (New York: Vintage Books, 1980), p. 222; C. S. Lewis, *The Problem of Pain* (New York: Macmillan, 1962), p. 24; T. Lewis, *Pain* (New York: Macmillan, 1942), pp. v–vii; G. Herbert, "Affliction," in *The Essential Herbert,* edited by A. Hecht (New York: Ecco Press, 1987), pp. 30–32; J. Donne, "Divine Meditations," in *John Donne: The Complete English Poems,* edited by A. J. Smith (New York: Penguin Books, 1972), p. 314.

8. E. J. Cassell, *The Nature of Suffering and the Goals of Medicine* (New York: Oxford University Press, 1991), pp. 30–33; J. Updike, "Pain," in *Facing Nature* (New York: Knopf, 1985), p. 54; J. Donne, "Fifth Meditation," in *Devotions upon Emergent Occasions,* edited by A. Raspa (Montreal: McGill-Queen's University Press, 1975), pp. 24–25.

9. H. K. Beecher, "Relationship of Significance of a Wound to the Pain Experienced," *Journal of the American Medical Association,* 1956, 61:1609–1615; H. K. Beecher, "The Measurement of Pain: A Prototype for the Quantitative Study of Subjective Responses," *Pharmacologic Reviews,* 1957, 9:59–209.

10. R. Melzack, "The Myth of Painless Childbirth," *Pain,* 1984, 19:321–337; K. L. Norr and others, "Explaining Pain and Enjoyment in Childbirth," *Journal of Health and Social Behavior,* 1977, 18: 260–265; I. P. M. Senden and others, "Labor Pain: A Comparison of Parturients in a Dutch and an American Teaching Hospital," *Obstetrics and Gynecology,* 1988, 71:541–544; B. Areskog, N. Uddenberg, and B. Kjessler, "Experience of Delivery in Women With and Without Antenatal Fear of Childbirth," *Gynecologic and Obstetric Investigation,* 1983, 16:1–12; R. Melzack and others, "Severity of Labour Pain: Influence of Physical as Well as Psychologic Variables," *Canadian Medical Association Journal,* 1984, 130:579–584.

11. L. M. M. Morrison, J. A. W. Wildsmith, and G. W. Ostheimer, "History of Pain Relief in Childbirth," in *Pain Relief and Anesthesia in Obstetrics,* edited by A. van Zundert and G. W. Ostheimer (New York: Churchill Livingstone, 1996), pp. 3–18; S. Hoffert, *Private Matters: American Attitudes Toward Childbearing and Infant Nur-*

ture in the Urban North, 1800–1860 (Urbana: University of Illinois Press, 1989), pp. 86–88; J. Cohen, "Doctor James Young Simpson, Rabbi Abraham DeSola, and Genesis, Chapter 3, Verse 16," *Obstetrics and Gynecology,* 1996, 88:895–898; "Text of Pope Pius' Address," *New York Times,* October 6, 1956.

INDEX

Page numbers in **boldface** refer to illustrations.